'Through his uncommonly broad experience and practice with the Alexander Technique, Feldenkrais Method, Hatha yoga, Rolfing and Hanna Somatics, Graeme Lynn has clarified the underlying principles that unify them. In this thoughtful and insightful analysis, Graeme effectively highlights their similarities and differences and provides the reader with interesting and practical exploratory exercises to deepen self-understanding. His book is a "must-read" for both experienced practitioners and also for those interested in improving the quality of functional life.'

– Al Wadleigh, Guild Certified Feldenkrais Practitioner,
owner of TheFeldenkraisStore.com

'Graeme Lynn is a somatic integrationist, melding the ideas of Moshe Feldenkrais, F.M. Alexander and Hatha yoga into a valuable resource for both the knowledgeable and the initiates among us. At the centre of this book lies learning, awareness and the basic principles of good self-organization. Enjoy this book and improve your health.'

– David Zemach-Bersin, senior Feldenkrais practitioner
and trainer, Feldenkrais Institute of New York, and
original student of Dr Moshe Feldenkrais

'Informative and insightful. If you are interested in how you move, breathe and think, this is the book for you. Lynn's wide-ranging experience and years of explorative study is clearly presented and delivered. Read it and learn more about yourself.'

– Carolyn Nicholls, AT teacher, head of training
at Brighton Alexander Technique College, and author of
Body, Breath and Being and The Posture Workbook

of related interest

Principles of the Alexander Technique
What it is, how it works, and what it can do for you
Second Edition
Jeremy Chance
ISBN 978 1 84819 128 0
eISBN 978 0 85701 105 3
Discovering Holistic Health

Meet Your Body
CORE Bodywork and Rolfing Tools to Release Bodymindcore Trauma
Noah Karrasch
Illustrated by Lovella Lindsey Norrell
ISBN 978 1 84819 016 0
eISBN 978 0 85701 000 1

Body Intelligence
Creating a New Environment
Second Edition
Ged Sumner
ISBN 978 1 84819 026 9
eIBSN 978 0 85701 011 7

AWAKENING SOMATIC INTELLIGENCE

Understanding, Learning and Practicing
the Alexander Technique,
Feldenkrais Method and Hatha Yoga

Graeme Lynn

Foreword by Michael D. Frederick

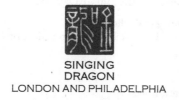

SINGING
DRAGON
LONDON AND PHILADELPHIA

First published in 2017
by Singing Dragon
an imprint of Jessica Kingsley Publishers
73 Collier Street
London N1 9BE, UK
and
400 Market Street, Suite 400
Philadelphia, PA 19106, USA

www.singingdragon.com

Library of Congress Cataloging in Publication Data
Names: Lynn, Graeme.
Title: Awakening somatic intelligence : understanding, learning & practicing the Alexander technique, Feldenkrais method & Hatha yoga / by Graeme Lynn.
Description: Wellesley, MA : Branden Books, [2015] | Includes bibliographical references and index.
Identifiers: LCCN 2015027370| ISBN 9780828325899 (pbk. : alk. paper) | ISBN 9780828325905 (e-book)
Subjects: LCSH: Mind and body therapies. | Alexander technique. | Feldenkrais method. | Hatha yoga.
Classification: LCC RC489.M53 L96 2015 | DDC 615.8/2--dc23 LC record available at https://urldefense.proofpoint.com/v2/url?u=https-3A__lccn.loc.gov_2015027370&d=BQIFAg&c=euGZstcaTDllvimEN8b7jXrwqOf-v5A_CdpgnVfiiMM&r=wyFYyPFjZJDRM7wbcP4G1xqgmAajjCPRiaHmleP9jKo&m=wojXY7QWBZDJqyQlLtVp5_LTxqRL468X1ItvWMaAk6w&s=91GYwKvxCaNX6ie-eBcvGurxiNaEMftO1j0MIxQ5JX4&e=

British Library Cataloguing in Publication Data
A CIP catalogue record for this book is available from the British Library

ISBN 978 1 84819 334 5
eISBN 978 0 85701 290 6

Printed and bound in Great Britain

Contents

THE NATURAL STATE

I am simply describing your ordinary state. You are functioning as awareness, then intelligence, associated with mind, emotion and body. In the Hindu tradition, the structure is described in terms of sheaths, the more outer being the physical, then the dimensions of natural energy and the emotional aspects of the person, then mind-forms and the psychic life, then this intelligence that observes it and that should be the controller of it, and, deeper than that, the awareness itself. The bodymind is described from the periphery to the centre as a collection of sheaths, with awareness at the center and the body and its field of activities at the periphery. This is simply an educational model to help people understand just how they are functioning in ordinary terms.

Adi Da Samraj

Monk: How then do we attain freedom?

Master: From the first, we have never been in bondage, and therefore there is no need to seek freedom. Just use the ways of freedom, act in freedom – this is indeed incomparable.

Zen story

Apollo

We'll never know his mythic head or blazing eyes,
And yet his torso, even now,
Stands here full charged with brilliance like a beacon
In which his ripened gaze, now turned down low,
Still shines in all its power.
Otherwise the curving breast could not so dazzle us
Nor could a smile descend
To those dark loins whence all of procreation flares.
Otherwise the stone would seem disfigured
In its falling from the lucent shoulders,
Not glisten like a lion's mane,
Would not from all its boundaries
Burst outwards like a star.
For here there is no place that is not seen.
I must transform my life.

Rainer Maria Rilke

Introduction

THE INFINITE NETWORK
OF POSSIBILITY

Imagine you are walking down a country road at dusk and, looking in the distance and through the dimming light, you see a darkened figure approaching you on foot. The shadows of the evening deepening into night conceal the clothes and person's features from the eye. How is it then you know and can recognize a friend?

You know because your friend and each of us *organize* ourselves in movement in a personally unique manner. This characteristic patterning derives in part from our inheritance but in larger measure from our experiential learning and we are active as that patterning, generally unconsciously, in everything we do.

What we inherit through our family of origin in physical terms remains a subject of research: organic strengths and weaknesses, bone structure and body type, facial features and so forth. The means whereby we learn and all of what we learn in terms of action patterns, movement and coordination are a more complex matter. In Ida Rolf's text, *The Integration of Human Structures*, she tells the story of a man who suffered severe injuries to a leg and his pelvis in the Second World War and who, though he lived and was otherwise healthy, consequently walked with a pronounced limp. After the war he married and had a son. Remarkably, before the boy had reached puberty he limped in the same way as his father.

This is not some weird and isolated aberration. We are each of us like that child in many complicated ways.

The ability of the human nervous system to learn, through which we adapt and change, is immense and subtle. We do not learn merely through imitation as in that story. Our physical development altogether, while guided genetically, is in part an open-ended process of functional learning. Our bodily expression of emotional character and fundamental beliefs is largely a matter of learning. How we adapt to and manifest ourselves physically in social interactions, work and play is learned. Also, as the mechanism reflexively responds to stress, injury, traumas of every kind, even disease, poor nutrition and surgery, how those responses are habituated is learning.

Stress, trauma, feeling, believing, imitation and development, in fact any experience or factor that instigates or involves a physical expression or response, which response is repeated, makes for learning – and specifically to our discussion here, *sensorimotor* learning. Most such learning occurs unconsciously and results in unconscious habits of *self-organization*, *moving* and *sensing*. As there are numberless learning possibilities so there are many ways for that process to go wrong.

The human structure, in terms of the skeleton and soft tissue, has a wide range of adaptability to patterns of *self-organization* or what Alexander called *use*. However, the chronic or recurrent aches and pains or worse, the rheumatic and arthritic conditions that many begin to suffer even in early adulthood, result from patterns of unconscious or habitual organization, or rather disorganization, which the structure can no longer tolerate. When stiffness, chronic tension or muscle contraction, chronic over-use or under-use, misalignment and sheering stresses, ischemia, hyper-mobility and so on go on too hard or too long pain begins and degenerative conditions result.

This deterioration can be reversed. Habitual patterns of poor self-organization and the consequent degeneration can be resolved through renewed sensorimotor learning. The Alexander Technique and the Feldenkrais Method represent the best in such ways of learning. Through these sophisticated learning methods a person becomes more sensitive to the quality of his or her movement and more integrated in movement and coordination. With time and practice, the sources of pain and decline are undone. The body is freed in action and regenerates.

There is a natural design of human function developed over the millions of years of our evolution in the context of gravity and each of us has an almost limitless capacity for learning in the form of our nervous system or natural intelligence. The Alexander Technique and the Feldenkrais Method take ingenious advantage of these facts and, through refined techniques of gentle manipulation,[1] facilitate learning of greater sensitivity to the physical self and an improved quality of movement, no matter what the problematic causes. Soon a person can more easily come to feel when an action is not harmonious with the structure and more readily find a coordination that is functionally competent and feels good. In this way one resolves problems before or after they have set in and comes to enjoy greater pleasure and agility in the body as the common experience of everyday life.

Age is not an obstacle to such renewal. The possible connections in the human nervous system outnumber the stars in the galaxy. This virtually infinite network of possibility is the source of our almost unlimited capacity to learn or relearn. We use only a portion of these connections even in our prime. Many so-called signs of ageing – pain, affliction and limitation – are often the results of complex learned patterns that can be undone and remade through the means used in these methods. The Alexander Technique and the Feldenkrais Method open new neural pathways through focused lessons that address the individual's needs and interests. These lessons provide concentrated sensorimotor experience relevant to the person's present state that he or she therefore welcomes and enjoys. This design and enjoyment make such learning interesting, usable, potent and more direct than the trial-and-error learning of childhood. This is how these methods can effectively resolve functional limitations and other problems that may arise in the course of our lives and so enhance the quality of life.

---

1   The word 'manipulation' here and throughout this book indicates movement, touch or handling as strategic interventions and does not imply brusqueness, force or coercion.

FREEDOM FROM REACTION

Michael D. Frederick

I first met Graeme Lynn more than twenty years ago at the beginning of his training in the Alexander Technique. As his path in the intervening years has followed a course similar to my own I hope that telling my story may offer a useful perspective on his synthesis of somatic disciplines.

I began my spiritual search under the tutelage of the iconoclastic teacher, J. G. Bennett, an ordinary man who, through his work in Gurdjieff's Fourth Way, had become extraordinary. The Fourth Way is a Western esoteric path whose goal is freedom from our dualistic patterning, where we are caught in the web of like and dislike, and the realization of Being in the senses of 'svadharma' and 'dharma'.

Gurdjieff saw that the traditional withdrawal from the world was not appropriate in this era and took the Sufi approach of 'being in the world but not of it'. One of Bennett's influential teachers was Shiva Puri Baba, a Buddhist whose first precept was to understand how the bodily mechanism works. With this essential understanding I began lessons in the Alexander Technique, about which I had heard much, and soon came to find the Technique revolutionary.

I was fascinated, not only because its principles struck me as true, but also because it works in the moment-to-moment of present action to release the individual into the natural state. By *subtracting* the interference of habitual patterning, what is left over is natural poise and good coordination, just as a sculptor works with marble by subtracting what is unnecessary and thereby rendering the work of art.

My interest in the Technique connected up remarkably with related teachings during that seminal period: the Gurdjieff work, Zen Buddhism, the wisdom of Jiddu Krishnamurti and yoga, all of which speak to freedom, wholeness, mindfulness in action and transcendence of the conditional self and social ego. I saw that the Technique offered me a fundamental practice to this end with its promise of freedom from compulsive and impulsive actions, from like and dislike and a ground for right living.

Walter Carrington, one of the great first-generation Alexander teachers, once said to me that the Technique is 'dead menial': that is, how you drive your car, work at the computer or drink a cup of tea – through mindfulness of such ordinary actions, the extraordinary quality of the present moment unfolds. The Technique connects me to this process.

After Alexander died in 1955, there was something of a diaspora of Alexander teachers. By the time I came to the Technique in the 1970s, the first-generation teachers were working independently. As they were then still in their prime I took the opportunity to take lessons from them and to get to know them all well.

I trained first with the Carringtons in London and then studied for years internationally with Marjorie Barstow, the first person to be certified by Alexander. Marj was innovative and original, a genuine debunker, challenging the habits and fears that I would hide behind. She questioned my boundaries in constructive ways that allowed me to move into greater self-understanding. The Carringtons' training made me a skilled practitioner. Marj's work took me a step further. She did not merely give an experience of freedom and lightness, which she did indeed do. She encouraged me and each student to be responsible for the quality of intention with respect to his or her every action. And when you were ready, she gave you the impulse to make the essence of the Work your own.

Having established relationships with the first-generation teachers, I was able to bring them together for the first of the International Alexander Technique Congresses, which continue today. When they came for that first Congress in 1986, because of their shared respect for and grasp of the spirit and essence of the Work, they were deeply connected to each other in a way that was profoundly moving for everyone. Although the Technique had developed since Alexander's time, as he had hoped, they still carried the spirit of the master.

So, what, you may ask, is that spirit? Well, do you ever get stressed or tense in your work or daily affairs? When you learn through the Technique to *un-do* that reaction that is causing the stress and tension, you find that spirit of lightness and ease that we seek in everyday life. With understanding and practice that lightness will enter into the rest of your life.

The Alexander Technique is a process of learning how to observe habits of action that create patterns of excessive tension in any activity – not only in your specialty in life, but in the way you carry out any ordinary activity. It is *psychophysical* re-education, the mindful undoing of unconscious habits.

There is a primitive reflex reaction in each of us, the fight-flight-freeze response that is activated in stressful situations – anytime there is a conflict between what is and what we feel should be. The Technique frees us fundamentally from that 'monkey in the cage' as the Buddhists describe it. And it works in real life, not as abstract philosophy.

Alexander brought what would otherwise remain mere philosophy into living. People can talk the talk and imagine they are making significant changes in their lives and growing. However, if they create unnecessary tension in themselves in their ordinary activities they are not actually aware of how their physical – or more correctly, psychophysical – habits conflict with their intentions at a basic level. Alexander made the foundation of real growth of the individual practical. He brought the Buddhist injunction of mindfulness into everyday activity but with a Western orientation independent of any esoteric teaching. As both Marjory Barlow, Alexander's niece, and Marjorie Barstow said to me, 'You are always going to lose your length. What you are learning is the art of regaining it.'

The many wonderful Alexander teachers with whom I have had the good fortune to work have instilled in me a profound *experiential* understanding of what psychophysical-emotional awareness is and how it allows us real choice in the present moment. It is straightforward and simple. And because of this simplicity and its potential for application in everyday life, which is today becoming so fragmented, Alexander's work is more relevant than ever.

To deepen my understanding of somatic work I began training in the Feldenkrais Method in the second American training in 1980 (the first American Feldenkrais training was in San Francisco a few years earlier). The Feldenkrais Method is sometimes compared to the Alexander Technique but really these methods live in different worlds. They can complement each other as Graeme has shown in his book, for the Feldenkrais Method, like the Alexander Technique, is a useful approach to sensorimotor learning. But where the Alexander Technique is a *subtle non-doing*, a letting go of the conditioned habit so that what is natural can emerge, the Feldenkrais Method is a *subtle doing*. The subtlety of this opens up the field of awareness and leads a person to a reduction of effort and improved function but it lacks the means to work within the unfolding moment and to practice in the now an improved use of the self. This is where the Alexander Technique begins.

Training in the Feldenkrais Method allowed me first to shed identification with Alexander orthodoxy and to see the Technique in a new light. It further allowed me more flexibility of thinking, letting fresh air in through the window as it were, thereby enhancing my teaching skills.

As with Hatha yoga, the Feldenkrais Method takes the range of movements beyond the daily round of sitting, standing, lying down, bending, reaching and walking. Based on developmental movement patterning, it is far more intelligent than repetitive exercises. After practicing yoga or working with Feldenkrais' Awareness Through Movement I have greater flexibility and flow in my body and central nervous system. Both these methods have value in this regard. Still I come back time and again to the Alexander Technique because it is about our psychophysical totality within the creative present.

In the Gurdjieff work they talk about entering the realm of 'all possibilities'. In the practice of the Technique, through the process of *inhibition* (meaning negation and subtraction, not repression), this potential exists, creating a space between the stimulus and the response, from which true creative action springs.

While teaching at the Krishnamurti school in Ojai, California in the late 1980s I began my study of yoga with Sonia Nelson and then, in India, under the tutelage of T. K. V. Desikachar, whose father, the renowned Sri T. Krishnamacharya, was the teacher of B. K. S. Iyengar and of Pattabhi Jois, the developer of Ashtanga yoga.

The study and practice of yoga are very much a part of my spiritual path. All my learning, in fact, is dedicated to the fundamental question, 'What is the sense and purpose of my existence?' Yoga, the Feldenkrais Method and the Alexander Technique help to clarify that purpose. They serve to integrate mind, body and feelings; they serve my right action by helping me to listen more; and most of all, they allow me to be kinder to other people. A paradox lies in the fact that these qualities of listening, kindness and integrity arise not as ends in themselves but as means within the unfolding moment. The process and end come together as one action.

Whenever I have had the chance to observe masters of these methods, I am most struck by their fundamental and enduring kindness. That, to me, is what these systems of psychophysical re-education are best intended to serve. And that takes study, understanding and practice. This book can help provide the basis for that.

Awakening Somatic Intelligence is a much-needed exploration of the Alexander Technique, the Feldenkrais Method and Hatha yoga and their compatibility and synergy. It gives interesting perspectives on these systems whose principles Graeme has clarified and elaborated. This book has made me think about my work in new ways, which is remarkable after having studied these methods for over thirty years. Graeme's use of language is especially stimulating and provocative. Gurdjieff, while writing his *magnum opus All and Everything*, used to write and rewrite, saying that he needed to 'bury the bone deeper': that is, we only make understanding our own when it is earned. Graeme is exploring this approach to writing. *Awakening Somatic Intelligence* is a thoughtful work about the Alexander Technique and psychophysical learning in general. It should be read several times.

Los Angeles, CA, USA
December 2008

THE NATURE OF WATER

In essence, the Alexander Technique is the purposive use of the mind in the context of the sensorimotor and biomechanical processes for the sake of optimal functioning. This book is an explanation and elaboration of that basic understanding. In any case, the most elaborate explanation is not a substitute for experiential practice.

Even so, I have explained the Technique from several perspectives that the reader may get different views of the subject. In telling Alexander's story of discovery we can join in his remarkable journey of self-understanding and mastery.

The description of the Technique's essentials, its organizing principles and the hierarchy of functions represent three models or ways in which to consider the method. I introduce the reader to simple ways of working on him- or herself and relate an introductory lesson and a not-so-introductory lesson that will exercise your somatic imagination and give you a feel for the practice in the context of the teacher–student paradigm. There follow some teaching remarks that highlight the kind of consideration involved in learning the Technique. We look at the manipulations used in the Alexander Technique and extend those traditional manipulations to Feldenkrais' Awareness Through Movement lessons and Hatha yoga *asanas* through which one can further evolve one's somatic ability. Finally I answer a variety of questions that can arise in the exploration of this work.

Thomas Hanna coined the term *somatic education* in the 1960s when he tied together the threads of philosophical and practical exploration undertaken by pioneers of the field that had until then been unnamed. Tom redefined the word 'soma' to refer to the 'inner experience of the sensorimotor process' and 'somatic' to mean 'pertaining to the body as perceived from within'.

Hanna said that, to understand somatic work and yourself as a somatic being, you have to 'walk through the looking glass' – because one's organization is a reflection of the use of the self, because somatic work will reflect your experience to you in a new way and because, like Alice, your experiences in the 'inner' world may require a revolutionary adaptation. Tom joked that the original mirror or looking glass is water.

The Technique and somatic work of any kind are best understood and practiced when one presumes that the self is psychophysical in nature. Though modern neurophysiology is founded on the materialist view, this view finds some acknowledgement in *The Fundamentals of Neurophysiology* (Schmidt 1985) where the author writes, 'When thought leads to action, the neurophysiologist is forced to accept that thinking can change the neuronal activity of the brain... Such conversion of thinking and intent into cortical impulse patterns remains, for the time being, far beyond the limits of our understanding.'

The sensorimotor process involves self-sensing, self-organization and the motor functions: movements, coordination, manipulations and the dynamic response to gravity. The *self-senses* are the senses that tell us about ourselves: balance, tissue tension, tissue pressure, felt movement, joint articulation and pain. *Self-organization* is the fact and manner that the whole body is 'shaped' by the mind (as agency) and as the physical self in the context of any action.

The sensorimotor nervous system has evolved as a cybernetic-like feedback circuit such that self-sensing impacts motor function and *vice versa*. And so, as self-sensing becomes truer, action becomes more harmonious and efficient; and as action becomes more harmonious and efficient, self-sensing becomes truer. The converse is also the case: when a person is suffering from a physical limitation they are therefore sensing themselves poorly; and if they are sensing themselves poorly they are moving and organizing their movement poorly. This understanding is at the foundation of somatic learning.

Some of Dr Wilfrid Barlow's studies suggest that the Technique encourages psycho-emotional maturation. One of Alexander's famous students, John Dewey, opined that the Technique serves a moralizing function. Alexander seemed to contradict such statements when he argued that the Technique would make a thief a better thief.

The Technique has demonstrated its effectiveness in improving the quality of life by improving functional ability. By freeing energy and attention otherwise bound in physical limitations and their results and by becoming thereby more effective, one comes to feel more self-assured and potent in the world. One gains greater functional autonomy and has more attention and energy for fulfilling one's interests.

In addition to those suffering a pain issue, those limited by inflexibility, a biomechanical disability, a breathing difficulty, a so-called postural problem, a performance barrier or any similar impairment will benefit from improved use of the self in action. A performance barrier could be in tennis, lawn bowling or running, making music, acting and so on. Some of Alexander's notable work was with golfers and actors though he never golfed and some say he could not act. The Technique has proved helpful in many specific areas of human endeavour and trouble: back, neck and shoulder pain; spinal injury; repetitive strain injury, frozen shoulder and tennis elbow; rehabilitation after stroke, injury and surgery; voice work; sports and fitness – improving coordination and suppleness and obviating injury; headache; high blood pressure; joint problems; anxiety and depression; stutter; asthma; horseback riding; the martial arts; and yoga. The Technique's benefits extend so broadly because, as Alexander explained, the use of the self is a universal constant in living (Alexander 2000). That is, our coordination of function and response to gravity are involved in our every activity.

Improving the use of the self must then benefit everything we do. We manifest as sense-based action. Our self-sensing and coordination are at the foundation of our health and adaptation to function and remain so throughout our lives. Anyone can benefit from the Technique because anyone can become more self-aware and coordinate movement more effectively. Furthermore, everyone can benefit, through generalizing to any activity, the use of attention, intelligence and intentionality that is essential to the practice of the Technique.

It is perhaps because of its fundamental contribution to our functional development and the education of the mental faculties in the context of function that Alexander wanted to see the Technique used in developmental learning. In fact, for some time he directed a small private school in England, then in the United States, where the Technique formed an essential part of the curriculum. Perhaps as it becomes obvious that the over-focus on intellectual and academic learning is detrimental to balanced maturation the Technique's adoption in schooling may be reconsidered.

The operative principles of the Alexander Technique are at the foundation of human improvement. The method provides us with a practical way to resolve our functional limitations. These familiar yet often inefficient patterns can result in disease, distress, harmful tension and unfulfilled potential. Alexander demonstrated that one can transcend these limitations and acquire exemplary coordination, alertness, greater freedom and a healthier use of ourselves. Since his original discoveries his work has received wide acclaim. Today the Technique is included in the curriculum of schools of music and the performing arts worldwide and as a supplement to conventional forms of healthcare typically when these modalities have failed. Conventional healthcare does not understand the fundamental influence of use on functioning and of functioning on bodily health and this is where the Alexander Technique begins.

Whether it is in artistic or athletic performance, physical health or in everyday life activities, the Technique's holistic approach demonstrates consistent benefits. The Technique is brilliant work developed by a genius pragmatist who, through a profound, painstaking and scientific study of and enquiry into his own sensorimotor processes and physical mechanics, rediscovered for himself and communicated to us all an effective method of physical renewal and discovered as well that health and healing are based in fundamental values and principles.

The Technique cannot be learned through reading about it. One will come to enjoy improved well-being only by exploring the dynamics of one's own action. This self-educative process will be aided immensely under the tutelage of a skilled teacher. Alexander said that what took him years to work out for himself can be accomplished in a few weeks with a good teacher.

This book is not therefore a substitute for the potent input of a teacher's educative handling and instruction. It is a thesis that may establish a good understanding of the Technique. If considered before and during lessons this study will, I hope, serve the progress of learning improved self-use both in everyday activities and in the exercise of specific arts and skills. I hope too that, as you work with this method, ideas presented here that you may not grasp at a first reading will become clear in your actual experience.

Summary Views

THE EVOLUTION OF A TECHNIQUE

Frederick Mathias Alexander was born in Tasmania in 1869, the first of a large family, and learned self-reliance early. As a youth he was troubled by respiratory difficulties which subsided in his high school years. When nearing graduation the headmaster withdrew Alexander from class to tutor him personally with the hopes that he might follow as headmaster. It has been suggested that the actual reason for separating Alexander from his classmates was that he asked too many questions.

However, Alexander was attracted to the stage and relocated to the mainland to pursue this interest. While working various jobs, he trained in acting. It was from this training that he learned at least one of the faulty habits of self-organization that he would unravel in the years to come. By the early 1890s he was having some success giving one-man performances at theatres around southern Australia.

After a few years pursuing his career in this fashion the problem that would change his life, but first ruin his vocational ambition, beset him: he repeatedly went hoarse on stage. In spite of frequent rests between shows as per his medical advice the problem worsened until Alexander realized that he could not continue without a real solution. Examination revealed nothing structurally wrong with the vocal apparatus that was the presumed source of the hoarseness. And the doctors' only remedy of rest did not actually resolve the problem.

This led Alexander to two conclusions, which are the backbone of the Technique. The first was that, since there was nothing wrong or diseased in his body, that is, nothing wrong with the *structure*, and since there was nothing inherently wrong or unhealthy with what he was doing, the *function*, acting and speaking, there must be something wrong with *how* he was doing what he was doing. Alexander came to call this 'how', in the most general sense, the *use* of himself. And because, as he discovered, use *organizes* function he realized that he was doing something wrong in his use and *self-organization* – the dynamic coordination of the whole of himself in action – which organization mediates use and function.

Second, Alexander realized that it was only himself who was responsible for the misuse, disorganization and dysfunction: responsible, both in the sense that it was he alone who was doing it and in the sense that it was he alone who could ever do anything to remedy it, because every action or reaction that I do is an action or reaction that only I myself do. He understood then that to seek passive treatment in response to any such use-, organization- or function-based problem must be inherently and ultimately ineffective; that he was responsible for and must change his own manner of action.

Alexander's story of the development of the Work in the chapter 'The Evolution of a Technique', in his third and most readable book, *The Use of the Self*, is amazing and profound. He began to observe himself reciting in front of an arrangement of mirrors. What he noticed as significant was that, in everyday actions but especially when declaiming or attempting anything stressful or demanding, he pulled his head down and back relative to his neck, 'decreased his stature' and narrowed his back. He came to notice that all of himself was involved in this pattern of contracting. In time he would come to notice that this self-contracting in the instigation and process of action was virtually universal to others and evident to the subtle observer in the process of every action.

In order then in a straightforward manner to correct this self-contracting reaction in the very process of initiating and carrying out a chosen action he determined to not do it anymore and instead to do the opposite. Thence came a profoundly disturbing discovery, which was that he could not not-do the contracting. Nor could he do the opposite in spite of his wish and intention to do so and even in spite of his *feeling* that he was doing so as he performed the action. He found that he could not directly and wilfully undo the self-contracting nor enact the opposite. In spite of feeling that he *was* doing what he meant to do the mirrors revealed that he continued to contract.

This must be emphasized: he visually observed using the mirrors – that is, perceived himself from the outside via the reliable visual sense – that he was doing other than what, on the inside, he kinaesthetically perceived that he was doing and what he meant to be doing, having determined what was best to do! In Alexander's own words: 'I was… suffering from a delusion that is practically universal…that because we are able to do what we "will to do" in acts that are habitual and involve familiar experiences, we shall be equally successful in doing what we "will to do" in acts which are contrary to our habit and therefore involve sensory experiences that are unfamiliar' (Alexander 2001).

Alexander was humbled and nonplussed. Perhaps not humbled.

He began exploring his movement anew and reconfirmed that, in the process of carrying out any action, all of the parts of himself and all of the functioning and organization of those parts are involved in every moment of action, and that the pattern of interference with the optimal use of himself equally involves all of himself, all of his parts and the organization and functioning of all of his parts. He realized that the pattern of interference was unconscious and habitual: that is, he was unable to sense it or to be responsible for it and it arose compulsively. The very habitual wrongness of his manner of doing and feeling was, he came to realize, an 'irresistible force' in determining the present manner of action and not to be easily overcome by a mere intention to do right.

In addition, it effectively undermined his ability to rightly sense what in fact he was doing and intended to do. This is so because, as was said earlier, the processes of self-sensing and movement are organized in the nervous system as in a cybernetic feedback loop wherein self-sensing informs movement and movement informs self-sensing.

Alexander recalled that he had cultivated some of his habits, thinking at the time that he was doing what was right and was able to wilfully do what he thought was right in the cultivation of those habits. As he wrote, 'the belief is very generally held that if only we are told what to do in order to correct a wrong, we can do it, and that if we *feel* we are doing it, all is well. All my experience, however, goes to show that this belief is a delusion' (Alexander 2001). Furthermore, he found that this cultivation of what were in fact negative habits – habits that undermined the optimal use of himself and were further causative of his limitation in function – seemed to be of greater force than merely unconsciously acquired habits and this because, in establishing such habits, one 'naturally' believes that one is doing right. Such habits thereby suffer the added emotional charge of 'the feeling of my being in the right', even though they are in fact ineffective, mal-coordinated or disorganized. Later he found that a greater force in undermining our will to change is our dependence on means that feel right and familiar based on how we habitually feel and function. When these means are found to be ineffective, obviously one must apply conscious intelligence to the present manner of action. Such is not always chosen: because of our dependence on these so-called 'natural' (that is, habitual) means; because we tend to focus on the goal of the action instead of the means and direction of the action; because the right means, that is to say, the optimal organization of the body in action, was never made explicit before Alexander's discovery; because we must go back to basics and begin learning movement fundamentals anew; and because, of course, we are lazy and passionate.

Alexander discovered that any action involves the whole body; that the organization of any necessarily whole-body action is controlled either cortically or subcortically, that is, consciously or habitually; and that the optimal manner of any action can be relearned only by conscious means. He discovered that the use of the bodily mechanism is epitomized in what he came to call *the primary control*, the unique human manner of organizing movement. The primary control is the 'shaping' or organization by the mind (as agency) as and of the core dynamic of the physical self, through which all human movement is expressed and which is inherent and implicit in every movement.

This so-called primary control involves the dynamic coordination of the relationship of the head with the neck and of the head–neck relationship with the back and, via the centre, with the rest of the body (the legs, arms and axial column) and via the pelvis and legs with the ground. This organization is sequential, instant and integrated and must be made conscious in order to obviate the manifestation of unconscious patterning or habit. Alexander (2001) said that messages must be 'freely and intentionally projected and energy so conducted to the right coordination of the mechanism' in order to revise the habitual organization.

As he began to gain a sense of and some small competence in this process he found himself confronted with a paradoxical obstacle. He found that his improved organization felt wrong!

In considering this he realized that, not only had he by tendency been depending on his own faulty self-sensing to determine how he was doing what he was doing – which accurate sensory determination is impossible because it is itself faulty – but, in addition, he was seeking to have sensations (in and of himself) that felt right in spite of the fact that they were completely unfamiliar!

Through remarkable persistence, he resolved this impasse by being more committed to 'doing right' than 'feeling right', *inhibiting* the habitual manner of organizing his movement, and at the same time *directing*, deliberately and step by step, what he had determined by rigorous investigation was the right present-time coordination for the optimal working of the mechanism. This involved keeping his interest first directed to that which he determined to be the best organization of the primary control for that step, and only secondarily directed to the apparent goal of the action and not at all to any familiar or unfamiliar feelings. This he called 'sticking to principle'.

The strategy that he devised was, while keeping that self-direction working, to change the intended action, delay it, not do it at all or do it anyway without attachment to its goal. By distracting himself thus from the *end* or goal of the chosen action and thereby weakening his compulsion thereto he indirectly strengthened his commitment to the present *means whereby* the goal is best achieved. Those present means are, at the psychical level, conscious intelligence applied to the action and, at the physical level, the organization of the movement or primary control, which is intrinsic to every movement and which defines the direction and thereby the goal of any movement.

In time, the habitual manner of doing and of feeling became obsolete through non-use and Alexander came to enjoy improved use and a greater feeling of well-being than he had previously experienced. In the years that followed he developed the instructional method through which he would teach this improved use to others.

Alexander's research and recovery of function took some nine years of work on himself. Some say it was many years beyond that before he completely understood and could clearly articulate what he was doing. (Indeed some say he never could clearly articulate what he was doing.) It took nearly forty years of private teaching before Alexander was persuaded that he could formally train others to teach what he was teaching and many more years before he allowed others to train teachers. In the intervening years, several of his assistants, Irene Tasker and Ethel Webb, and his brother, Albert Rudolph Alexander, apprenticed to F.M., as Alexander was called, and learned to teach the Technique. But it wasn't until 1931 that Alexander began the first formal course wherein he would train as teachers a group of about a dozen interested men and women who had been taking private lessons with him.

During and after this initial period of exploration in the 1890s Alexander began teaching what he had learned to others, especially those in the theatre. At first, he told people what to do but he soon found that such verbal instruction was ineffective. It was thus that he happened upon the use of his hands to manually organize a person's movement and coordination, an intervention that makes it unnecessary for a person to discover through the same painstaking research as Alexander himself the optimal coordination of the mechanism. For many years this kind of teaching by handling was unique to the Work.

Although in the beginning he was known as 'the breathing man' because of the impact on the quality of respiration afforded by the method he soon found that his technique had wider applications.

As his success grew he was inspired to seek his fame and fortune in the capital of the then Empire and was encouraged by friends and associates, especially and remarkably in the medical field, who were referring their difficult patients to him and recommending his work highly. In Alexander's flamboyant style, he paid for his passage to England from the winnings of a horseracing bet.

For many years, he taught privately in London and, during the war years, on the eastern seaboard of America. His success grew but then, as now, the Technique confronted medical bias and the scientific materialist paradigm. The principles of the Technique challenge some of our strongly held beliefs about the nature of reality in general and about ourselves in particular. It is a subtle process both in terms of its conceptual foundations and in terms of the physical changes induced. And it requires commitment and patience to stay with the process of unknowing and change.

Alexander wrote four books wherein he explained the profound and useful nature and practice of the Work. One can gather from the personal force evident in these books that he knew the cultural bias he confronted. Alexander never lost his passion for the Work and taught until only a few weeks before his death in 1955 at the age of eighty-six.

He was not only a passionate man but evidently a delightful companion and friend. He supported a large extended family throughout his life and had a deep love for children and a gentle respect for those who came under his care. He was something of a storyteller and trickster and carried a love for theatre, equestrianism and gambling to his grave. Michael Bloch's excellent and non-idolatrous biography, *FM: The Life of Frederick Matthias Alexander*, describes a man of maturity and of great emotional and functional capacity, far ahead of his time in his thinking, attitudes and conduct.

Alexander went through three phases of communicating the method, which produced three generations of teachers with different styles of teaching. The first phase may have resulted from his own undeveloped handling skills and from the way Alexander had worked out the method for himself, which relied mostly on refusing to respond in an habitual manner to a stimulus, whether an impulse from within or a response to something from without. Thus, the emphasis of teachers trained in the early years was on the pupil's *inhibition* or *non-doing* of the habitual reaction and less on the teacher's manipulation – a skill that takes years to refine.

Later teachers became more affirmative in their handling. Perhaps the people Alexander worked with in the post-Victorian era were less bodily self-aware than now and generally more held and therefore required stronger stimuli to awaken their self-sensing. Perhaps it was because Alexander himself found that he could get faster changes in his pupils if he instructed them less in inhibition and instead gave them repeated clear experiences of a better organization of the primary control and of themselves altogether.

It is interesting to note that, in the early years of my own training, my first teacher was quite firm in his manual direction and that, as I improved in my use, his manipulation became more subtle.

In 1949, Alexander suffered a stroke. After this incident, from which he recovered well, his strength was compromised but he continued teaching and training teachers. In this phase of his work his manipulation became subtler because of his reduced strength and the results he achieved with his pupils seemed greater. In the case of teachers trained in this way the good use of the teacher and the greater refinement of the manipulation itself combined to benefit both the pupil and the teacher in the best way.

In the United States, A.R. Alexander and Marjorie Barstow promoted the work after the Second World War. Barstow had been certified by F.M. in his first training course. A.R. had suffered a devastating back injury in a fall from a horse and taught from a chair. Barstow developed a method of teaching the Technique in groups. It is possible that the 'doing and feeling' form of the Technique taught by some American teachers today was an historical result of the more hands-off styles of teaching necessitated by A.R.'s condition and created by Barstow's group developments. ('Doing and feeling' is shorthand for performing an action, such as sitting, standing or walking, and feeling how and what one feels in the context of one's growing sense of the primary control.) In the years following Alexander's death in 1955, the Technique's popularity waned. Then, with the advent of the human potential movement and given the Technique's place as a seminal discipline of the holistic paradigm the Technique has found a new following and is now recognized as an effective method for transcending physical limitations and improving function.

At this time there are training programs worldwide. Most are affiliated with several certifying organizations. Certification generally requires fifteen hundred hours of training over three years and the imprimatur of the school's educational director.

The Technique is taught privately and in groups. Although some still argue about it, undoubtedly the more effective means whereby improved use is learned, as Alexander himself discovered at the start of his teaching, is the direct transmission from teacher to pupil. Alexander typically began pupils with thirty lessons, five lessons a week for six weeks. This intensity of lessons is unfortunately hardly possible except among the most interested and well-to-do. Still this standard remains an excellent ideal. This is because our habits of misuse are, in general, deep-rooted and are 'practiced' at all times we do not apply a greater force for change in the forms of self-awareness and intelligence in action. Like any learning, whether it is riding a bicycle or playing a musical instrument and so on, the greater frequency of practice speeds the process of mastery. In this work, of course, the instrument one is seeking to master is oneself.

Today one can find teachers in most cities worldwide. There are national societies of teachers of the Alexander Technique in many countries, which maintain standards of training and practice.

The Alexander Technique is a unique and effective method of psychophysical or somatic education, founded on the principles and values of self-awareness, embodiment, holism, learning and freedom or the transcendence of habit. These principles, which emerged from Alexander's profound practical self-exploration, establish the Alexander Technique as good philosophy and a primary discipline of good health. Because of its fundamental principles it has implications that exceed its humble purposes. Alexander's work has had a positive impact, not only in ordinary people's active lives, but also through its influence on many renowned scientists, educators, thinkers, psychologists and artists of the twentieth century.

ESSENTIALS OF THE WORK

Alexander said that, in this method, we are duplicating what happens in Nature when conditions are right, only we're learning to do it consciously. It is obvious that what makes the Technique a potent tool for growth is this use of conscious intelligence relative to function. What makes Alexander's discovery extraordinary was his persistence in the face of the paradox of unconsciousness with respect to the use of himself. This unconsciousness of an unnatural reaction pattern resulted in the frustration of intention.

Alexander's investigation was a persistent application of his intelligence or, as he said, his reason, to the understanding of his thinking *vis-à-vis* his action. From this came the fundamentals of the Technique: freedom; learning; the integrity of the physical mechanism, of sensorimotor functioning and of the human event altogether as a psychophysical process; the universality of self-contracting habits and the resultant unreliability of self-sensing and consequent relative ineffectiveness of action; the fact of a senior integrating function; and the establishment of good habits of use for optimal functioning.

These good habits are: self-awareness or present-time attention[1] to what Alexander called the *means whereby* of any action – and thus

---

1   'If the various functional levels of the body-mind can be "rightly" perceived and (most fundamentally) understood, then the key to each stage of spiritual practice is Revealed. This "right" perception and most fundamental understanding is already suggested by the traditional names for the functional levels (or "sheaths" or "coverings" or "superimpositions" on Consciousness) represented by the body-mind.

'The "gross body" or physical body is "*annamayakosha*" or the "food sheath".

'The "subtle body" or the "internal" personality (or group of functions) is made of three fundamental parts. The first (which may be contacted inwardly but the relinquishment of *end-gaining*; intentional self-direction; and self-responsibility in the forms of self-understanding and choice: understanding that one is the agent of one's own actions for good or ill and choosing in present time an intelligent manner of action.

FREEDOM

Freedom is both the means and purpose of the Technique. Attention or the faculty of observation, intelligence and intention are, by their nature, free of mental, emotional and physical habit. Freedom in this sense is inherent: limitation is what we add accidentally, reactively, naively, unconsciously, by imitation, for emotional gains and so on. We can relocate our inherent freedom by the primary intentional act of not reacting habitually. Attention and intelligence give us the means to understand our habits of action. Intention as *inhibition* is the means of undoing the habits and as *direction*, of organizing a new manner of action.

---

which is really surrounding the "gross body") is "*pranamayakosha*" (or the "pranic sheath", or the "body of personal life-energy"). The second is "*manomayakosha*" (or the "sheath of lower mind"). The lower mind includes the conscious, subconscious and the unconscious minds. The functional activity of the lower mind (or brain-mind) is generated from a position that stands above and senior to the "pranic body". The third (and most senior) part of the "subtle body" is "*vijnanamayakosha*" (the "sheath of higher mind" or the "sheath of intellect"). At the core of the higher mind is the central will and discriminative (and naturally observant) intelligence of the conditional ego-"I" or limited self, and its functional activity is generated from a position that stands above and is central and senior to the "sheath of lower mind".

'Finally, there is "*anandamayakosha*", the "sheath of conditional bliss" or "causal body", which is the causative root of conditional selfhood. The "causal body" is associated with the right side of the heart (which is itself the Ultimate Passageway to Transcendental Spiritual Self-Consciousness)' (Samraj 1999).

The 'attention' or 'awareness' applied in the Alexander Technique and the Feldenkrais Method is not the root attention that Adi Da says is the essence of the 'causal body' nor Transcendental consciousness but the natural function of observation that, like intelligence or the intellect and intention or the will, is a core function of *vijnanamayakosha*.

THE FOUNDATION OF LEARNING

Learning, as Alexander said, requires the acceptance in one's experience of the unknown and, as Feldenkrais remarked, is realized in the ability to respond in new ways. Inhibition, the non-doing of the habitual reaction to a stimulus, is the means whereby one may discover something new. As Alexander (2001) wrote, 'by this primary act of prevention, the way is left clear to learn a new direction of use of the mechanisms, which would constitute the means whereby a person would in time be able to use the mechanism as an integrated unity'. Non-doing of the old allows for learning a new adaptation for which we have a virtually limitless capacity.

Learning is made direct in an Alexander lesson via a sensorimotor learning strategy called the principle of reafference. The use of this principle makes sensorimotor learning more effective because it happens that, when the learner makes some voluntary use of his or her musculature while the teacher facilitates an improved manner of movement, new adaptation is more readily achieved.

THE INTEGRITY OF THE PHYSICAL MECHANISM

As the song goes, 'the head bone's connected to the neck bone, the neck bone's connected to the backbone', and so forth. Our functional integration is more complex than the song would suggest. One can look at any action and see a collaboration of effort and organization with more or less of every part involved in the action. The Technique is purposed to consciously harmonize that integration via the primary control, the way of responding as the whole person from inside to out.

RELAXATION

In the beginning of his teaching Alexander instructed people to relax the neck, the back and so on, and discovered that the word 'relax' was associated in people's minds with making oneself heavy and tended to produce collapse. One of the interim goals of practice of the Technique is, in contrast, alertness and lightness of feeling and action.

At the same time, one is seeking to accomplish the tasks of life with relaxed effectiveness, free of extraneous effort. By having energy and attention freed from chronic patterns one becomes more relaxed, aware and effective.

A limitation in relaxation practices such as massage,/ some forms of meditation and so on is that, if used as remedies for chronic tension and distress, one is not learning a better present-time response to stressors and challenges. In the Technique, one is learning to practice relaxation in the context of every action.

THE HUMAN PROCESS AS AN INTEGRATED PSYCHOPHYSICAL EVENT

It was perhaps Alexander in the West who first suggested the fact of psychophysical integrity. In *The Use of the Self*, he wrote, 'when I began my investigation, I...conceived of the "body" and "mind" as separate parts of the same organism, and consequently believed that human ills, difficulties and shortcomings could be classified as either "mental" or "physical" and dealt with on specifically "mental" or specifically "physical" lines. My practical experiences, however, have led me to abandon this point of view... [T]he Technique...is based on the opposite conception, namely, that it is impossible to separate the "mental" and "physical" in any form of human activity' (Alexander 2001).

This revolutionary perspective has yet to be understood in Western culture though Alexander convincingly argues for it. In failing to understand that every action is psychophysical in nature a person will not notice that how and what he or she is thinking and presuming is influencing the quality of his or her actions and may look in the wrong place for the source of suffering.

Although it is impossible to adequately describe subjective experience even as it pertains to physical activity, in terms of the response to any event in our experience, some awareness is involved, usually some obvious interest, intention or desire, and some measure of intelligence or thought. As higher-order somatic events their existence is evident but not definable.

A new-age argument is that the body and mind are one, whatever that might mean. That is not what Alexander is suggesting any more than that the wall and the floor of a room are one: the wall bounds the room, the floor supports the contents; the mind thinks, the body moves. One can distinguish a thought from a movement even if the thought stimulates the movement.

In Daniel Goldman's book, *Emotional Intelligence*, studies are reported of people who, lacking emotional affect due to damage to the brain centres that mediate emotion, cannot make a decision to act. This validation of integration *vis-à-vis* the emotional component of action goes beyond the scope of the Alexander Technique but further confirms scientifically the integration of human function that Alexander discovered experientially.

THE UNIVERSALITY OF SELF-CONTRACTING HABITS OF MOVEMENT, COORDINATION AND ACTURE[2] AND THE RESULTANT UNRELIABILITY OF SELF-SENSING AND VICIOUS SPIRAL OF INCREASINGLY UNRELIABLE AND INEFFECTIVE FUNCTION

Alexander observed that poor use was endemic. Poor use or habits of action begin with faulty reaction patterns (brought on by reflex responses to stress, injury, surgery, disease and traumas of every kind, and by lifestyle habits, faulty development and imitation in youth, and in the physical manifestation of emotional patterning, character strategies, fundamental beliefs, even poor nutrition, and indeed by any

---

2   Feldenkrais coined this clever term. 'Acture' describes the ongoing dynamic response to gravity, which can be distinguished both inwardly and outwardly from movement, and differentiates this dynamic response to gravity from the *denotation* of the word 'posture', and from that word's *connotations* of stasis, positioning and rigidity, which concepts fail to grasp the anti-gravity response as a dynamic function. I will use the term 'actural dynamic' to describe the dynamic, responsive, 'anti-gravity' organization of human movement when supported via the upward thrust of the trunk (and legs) through any present-time moment of movement.

factors that repeatedly or strongly stimulate reaction) and because of the inextricable effect of action on self-sensing, deficient patterns of self-sensing. Deterioration in function then follows.

In general we must be convinced we are responsible for the results of our actions in terms of pain, disease processes or diminished sensitivity and for the relative ineffectiveness of our actions and frustration of our intentions.

An interesting way to illustrate the generation of faulty habits is to describe how to cook a frog. Everyone has seen how frogs can sit around and do nothing all day wasting their lives. If you place such a lazy frog in tepid water so that it is comfortable in the manner to which it has grown accustomed in its habitual laziness and if you raise the temperature slowly enough, its sensory mechanisms *cannot* register the gradual change in temperature and eventually you can bring the water to a boil and cook the frog. Its ability to sense changes in heat can be bypassed if the temperature changes are gradual enough. This is because sensory acuity works quantitatively not continuously.

As it is with frogs so it is with us. For instance, if you are carrying a forty-pound load, it is perceptually impossible to feel the addition of the weight of something less than a pound. The sensory organs embedded in the tendons, which determine the perception of weight, are not evolved to be sensitive to less than about a 2.5 percent change in the measure of the stimulus. However, if you are carrying, say, a two-pound stone, the addition of something weighing about an ounce *can* be noticed. All of the senses register changes according to a specific ratio of smallest noticeable differences. This is the *Weber–Fechner* principle.

If, in our reactions to stressors, limitations are introduced into our function, those changes may be so slight that they cannot be noticed. Those limitations then become a part of a new 'normal', which feels the same as the old 'normal'. We don't, because we can't, notice the spiral of poor and poorer habits. This process may continue until we find ourselves in a situation like Alexander: a conflict between intention and result. Or we begin to suffer unexplained pain, affliction and limitation. This is how the straw broke the camel's back, how

Alexander lost his voice, how accidents and ailments seem to appear suddenly.

The counterpart to this degeneration is the difficulty in making changes for the better. I travel by bicycle and generally wear a backpack so that I usually have the kinaesthetic experience of at least a small weight on my back. The other day riding home, I passed the local cinema and noticed a film I wanted to see on the matinee. I rode home for a snack then went back to the cinema without my backpack. Part way there I began to feel that something was wrong until I remembered that I was without my pack and realized that I was missing the kinaesthetic experience of the weight of the pack on my back.

However you characteristically or habitually organize your movement gives you constant kinaesthetic experiences of yourself a hundred and sixty-eight hours a week. Imagine if those experiences suddenly vanished. The nervous system would move to recreate those familiar kinaesthetic experiences by stimulating the very complex of muscular contractions that make for your habitual organization and that are the source both of your familiar 'self-identity' and of the somatic problems you may be suffering. This is why improvements are difficult to make and sustain. It is the essence of the force of habit.

The ramifications of this go further. We communicate our emotions and our character altogether to ourselves and to others verbally via our thinking and words, but also muscularly through our kinaesthesia and body language. If the characteristic muscular patterns that define us and the consequent kinaesthesia cannot be changed readily, so our emotional and character patterning will tend to remain in fixed patterns of action and expression.

THE FOURTEEN SENSES

Everybody knows that eyes see, ears hear, the skin senses surfaces and feels cold and heat, the tongue tastes and the nose smells. (Some blind people, as it happens, can 'visually' sense verticals and horizontals because of a secondary neural pathway, which we all have, distinct from the optic nerves that carry the impulses related to colours and black and white. This sense is called 'blind sight'.) The six self-senses, or kinaesthetic and proprioceptive senses, are balance, joint articulation, felt movement, tissue pressure, tissue tension and pain. Few of us consciously consider these as sensory in nature. Even fewer realize that deficiencies in such self-sensing deteriorate the quality of our actions and our experience of ourselves.

The vestibular apparatus, the sensory receptors for balance, are located in the semi-circular canals of the inner ears. There are receptors for balance concentrated in the neck, the back and the soles of the feet and many sparsely distributed throughout the body. The joint capsule receptors are sense organs that inform the brain about the articulation of the joints. These sensations provide the main basis for the perception of our skeletons and shape altogether. The sense organs called muscle spindles, embedded in every muscle, inform us that, how and how fast the muscles are moving and thereby how the bones are moving. They provide the sense and perception of movement and of the motion of the body through space. The pressure receptors, embedded in the connective tissue throughout the body, tell us of the measure of compression within or pressure on the myofascia, the muscle and connective tissue network. The Golgi stretch receptors, located in the tendons that attach muscles to bones, register the degree of tension in the tendons and so significantly inform the perception of the relative contraction of the associated musculature. Free nerve endings act as pain receptors. These register the presence of excess foreign substances in the tissues, especially of lactic acid, the by-product of chronic muscle 'tension'. They also register strain from excessive compression or stretching in the tissues and, of course, inflammation and tissue damage.

The re-education of these senses in the Alexander Technique affords us a better overall and more detailed sense of ourselves and so the potential, because of the cybernetic-like interrelation between self-sensing and motor function, for an improved quality of movement.

The nervous system receives sensory information from the body. If self-sensing is faulty or deficient, then the consequent actions will be relatively ineffective or dis-integrated.

Equally, if actions are ineffective, then the sensory information will be deficient.[3] The combined effect of awareness, intelligence and intention in the context of the sensorimotor process provides a means of refinement and re-education of function.

THE FACT OF A SENIOR ORGANIZING FUNCTION

The *primary control*[4] involves the dynamics and coordination of the relationship of the head with the neck and of the head–neck relationship with the back and, via the centre, with the rest of the body and via the pelvis and legs with the ground. By rightly organizing the primary control, physical action conforms to the mechanical requirements of the structure for movement and of the structure's gravitational relationship with the earth.

---

3   There is an unfathomably vast number of sensory data converging upon the brain in any moment. According to the so-called Gate Theory, only certain information is passed via this proposed gate to the central nervous system. The determining factor in this selectivity may be what is judged by a higher-order function, such as need, interest, intention or desire, as most valuable to the person. This may mediate the sensory information and guide the motor response.

4   Although Alexander himself did not state it, the primary control is best understood as being psychophysical in nature in that it is the 'shaping' or organizing by the *mind* as and of the *physical mechanism*: that is, it is the 'mental' action of intending-relaxing of the self-contracting patterns of the body and, springing from that release and based on feedback from self-sensing, the intending-directing of the organization ('all at once, one after another') of the mechanism in movement in the actural dynamic through any moment of time; and it is the (sequential, instant and integrated) 'physical' organization itself of that movement. In Alexander's language it is a 'certain' organization; Patrick MacDonald, one of Alexander's early protégés who developed his own style of teaching, might have said a 'proper' organization. Anyway, it is the native, natural or uncomplicated organization of any present movement of the body in the actural dynamic through a moment of time. In general, I will be using the term in those terms.

Control might suggest to some an 'agent' 'inside' 'in control', none of which three concepts is implied in the Technique. For a perfect understanding of dualism and non-dualism, see 'God-Talk, Real-God-Realization, Most Perfect Divine Self-Awakening and The Seven Possible Stages of Life' in *The Gnosticon* by Avatar Adi Da Samraj.

Some presume that the primary control is a postulate peculiar to the Technique or that it is a separate thing or function in the human being that may or may not be located somewhere or somehow and that one can choose to use or not use it, accept or reject it.

To clarify this misunderstanding, picture a moving snake. That distinct manner of movement is not a process or thing in subtle form but rather the way or manner of moving that snakes exhibit, which worms in contrast, whose shape is similar to snakes, do not. The human manner of organizing movement is one that is natural to human carriage, which is obviously different from that of a bird or ape. A teacher of the Technique understands and communicates manually that way of organizing movement: it involves directions, a sequential organization of the mechanism, a play of forces, a dynamic potential and a relativity of parts. It can be perceived both inwardly, which perception is the basis of the ability to work on oneself, and outwardly, the basis for hands-on manipulation.

The primary control cannot be separated from any present-time action. It is the present and prior organization or 'shaping' of this and every next moment of action.

THE IMPORTANCE OF GOOD HABITS

Good habits of mind and action make life easier. The establishment of good habits supports freedom in action, which is the essence and goal of the Technique. The apparent line between 'conscious constructive control', as Alexander described it, and what one might call 'unconscious constructive control' is vague as the improved manner of action consciously and freely learned via the Technique is always accessible to conscious reconsideration and adjustment.

STRUCTURE, FUNCTION, SELF-ORGANIZATION AND USE

What Ida Rolf called the *organ of structure* is the three-dimensional connective tissue network interwoven throughout the body, surface to core. Rolf found that this soft collagen-rich colloidal tissue can be molded by direct deep 'manipulation', which unique form of manipulation is the essence of the manual therapy she developed called *structural bodywork*. Our basic *structure* is given at birth and adapts in response to *function*. Function includes the developmental processes and all the kinds of actions performed, which actions are accomplished by the work of muscles. The structure both determines what kind of functions are afforded and is shaped by what and how functions are performed. *Use* involves the mental processes of awareness (attention or interested observation), intelligence and intention. The term 'use' can also be applied to the coordination of the structure, which is better described as *organization* or *self-organization*. The Technique then is a technology of *use* in its application to *organization* and sensorimotor and biomechanical *function* and to the coordination and mechanics of the *structure*. The human structure's unique orientation to gravity determines the nature of the primary control.

Improving use improves function, which in time improves the quality and form of the structure. Conversely, by improving structure one can make way for improved function. By improving structure or function, one frees energy and attention for better use.

The Technique is a generalist approach that applies the mental faculties primarily to organizing function. Improvements in function and structure emerge spontaneously. Problems with pain, which is caused by stress upon the structure, disappear as function improves. Weakness of muscular support mechanisms, build-up of fat tissue and other structural issues will tend to resolve as competence improves in function and self-organization.

Without improving use the address to structure will tend to be limited in its long-term effects, something practitioners of Rolfing have discovered in their work. Reorganizing structure through manipulation of the connective tissue network allows for better function, but without the conscious exploitation of that improved functioning the habitual patterns tend to recreate the adhesions. While Rolfing can be necessary and effective in many cases where adhesions in the tissues are significant, the benefits of ordinary massage and chiropractic, except in the hands of exceptional practitioners, are limited.

Use is the measure of intelligence and freedom brought to the organization of any moment of action. In methods that work to improve function the understanding of use is lacking as is an organizing *motor concept*, the primary control, the vital importance of which core dynamic emerges from an understanding of the coordination of the structure in the actural dynamic. Students of such methods are without a means of moment-to-moment conscious practice and depend on unconscious governance for their present-time sense of competent action, the very unconscious governance that undermined Alexander's initial attempts to change his manner of action. Such unconscious governance will tend to be inadequate until the ineffective patterns of action that bring a person to such work are made conscious and resolved.

The primary control allows for the limitations of attention and provides a 'feed-forward sensorimotor image', which is functional, present-time and accessible and by which to assess the quality of one's use. In the Alexander lesson this 'image' is transmitted by the teacher again and again and the improving organization allows the person to project its realization in action.

The action of present-time consciousness with respect to the physical mechanism is primary and improving function emerges through one's conscious presence. The Technique thus serves as a meta-practice with respect to other somatic methods.

Structure consists of the connective tissue network of the body as the medium of the muscles. Soft connective tissue is a unique substance in the body, making up a remarkable 25–35 per cent of body mass. It consists mainly of a ground substance and string-like microfibres called collagen, which 'float' in the ground substance in colloidal suspension rather like strips of lemon zest in a jelly. Depending on the density, combination and organization of these principal constituents, soft connective tissue can be tendons, ligaments or fascia. It can be loose or dense with collagen; and it can consist of disorganized or organized collagen. If organized and dense, the collagen can be crosshatched as in a ligament or aligned as in a tendon. If it consists mainly of ground substance and disorganized collagen it is fascia. Fascia works in a remarkable variety of ways depending on the proportions of its prime constituents: like a lubricant to allow tissues to slide upon each other; like liquid glue to keep the parts intact; and like clay to shape the physical form. Fascia invests every tissue in the body down to the microscopic units of muscle. It is the ocean in which all the other bodily tissues are suspended.

Connective tissue, whether it is bone, ligament, tendon or fascia, adapts to the stresses or forces to which it is subjected. Movements and the response to gravity are the forces that form and 'inform' all connective tissue causing adaptive changes in its looseness, alignment, organization, fluidity and strength. Such changes involve, first, the fascia. Bone, cartilage, ligaments and tendons can and do change with time but it is the fascia that adapts most readily. Habituated functional and 'postural' patterns over time cause it to become stiff just as jelly hardens if left to dry on a countertop. Dense adhesions may result which cannot be readily resolved with functional work only. When adhesions are fixed, structural bodywork, powerful contraction of the related musculature, stretching or toning may be required for quicker changes, even for any real change at all.

When one views one's shape in terms of its divergence from 'ideal lines', those divergences or anomalies can be caused by what the musculature is doing in the present – which doing can be potentially resolved at any moment by undoing or changing the doing – or by what the musculature has been doing over time that has shaped and now fixed or patterned the fascia and other connective tissue.

Because structure adapts to function and self-organization it can be viewed as crystallized function. If the function is chronic then the adaptations of the structure can be binding. We have all seen the elderly in whom the bones of the ribcage and spine are misshapen by the long-standing crunching of the trunk. Scoliosis can produce similar distortions of the ribs and spine. Chronically raised shoulders from anxiety can shorten the collarbones and flatten and narrow the ribcage. Many such distortions of form are evident on every street in every city in the world. Less exaggerated patterns can cause adaptations of the soft connective tissue resulting in inflexibility, aches and pains, misalignment and shearing stresses, imbalance of forces through the frame causing joint inflammation and so forth.

Sometimes structural bodywork is a useful or necessary preliminary or adjunct to somatic work. If the structural distortions are very limiting, direct work on the structure may be needed to elicit some movement where there is little or none. Without some perceivable movement made available by such work, the person may have too much difficulty sensing themselves to make functional work practicable. On the other hand, during Alexander's first training course, one day he announced to the class that his best student had just entered the offices for a lesson. Everyone rushed out of the training room to see the star pupil only to find a bent-up old lady waiting.

YOGA: STRUCTURE AND FUNCTION

Yoga is one of the orthodox systems of Indian philosophy, systematized by Patanjali. Yoga is so called because it seeks, by skilful means, to unite or yoke the individual soul or *atman* to *Paramatma*, the Supreme Self of which the *atman* is conceived to be a part. Patanjali enumerates these means as the eight advancing limbs (*ashtanga*) of yoga: *yama* (moral commandments: non-violence, truth, non-stealing, continence, non-coveting); *niyama* (self-purification: purity, contentment, austerity, study, devotion); *asana* (posture); *pranayama* (control of the breath); *pratyahara* (freedom from sense-based mind); *dharana* (concentration); *dhyana* (meditation); and *samadhi* (Realization). Yoga is typically limited to the practice of *asanas* or poses.

From a musculoskeletal point of view, a typical *asana* requires the 'stretching' of certain muscles and sometimes the relatively strong contraction of the antagonistic muscles. (The triceps muscle, which straightens the elbow, is the antagonist of the biceps muscle, which bends the elbow, and *vice versa*: the biceps is the antagonist of the triceps.) In fact, it is impossible to stretch a muscle. The chemical bonds that shorten muscles have the strength of tensile steel. In the stretch assumed in a yoga pose, it is the tendons and ligaments – the structure of the body therefore – that may be stretched. The stretch to the tendons stimulates the embedded Golgi stretch receptors whose information sent to the brain may cause a reflexive release of the muscles that are attached by those tendons to the bone. (In a forward bending pose, for instance, the dozens of tendons associated with the paraspinal musculature from head to tail are put on stretch, stimulating that musculature to release and allow the back to lengthen.) A strong contraction of muscles can strengthen the muscles as any exercise does but it also 'loudly' informs the nervous system of the organization of those muscles as per the Weber–Fechner principle.

In addition, the musculature antagonistic to the contracted musculature releases through a spinal cord reflex called reciprocal inhibition. For example, when you contract the biceps muscle, the triceps muscle reflexively releases to allow the bending of the elbow and, again, *vice versa*: contracting the triceps muscle inhibits the biceps muscle and allows the arm to straighten. Like the relaxation of muscles attached to stretched tendons and the sensory information with respect to the organization of the musculature for the pose, the muscular release effected by reciprocal inhibition is a functional event when there is attention to the release. The pose also stretches and aligns the tendons, ligaments and the fascia investing the muscles. This stretching and alignment is a structural change. Thus, an *asana* changes structure, by stretching and aligning connective tissue, and it potentially changes function: first, through the information provided by the muscular contractions; second, through the inhibition of the antagonistic muscles; and third, through the reflexive release of those muscles stimulated by the stretching of their associated tendons.

BASIC COORDINATION

In this practice we re-establish the natural manner of action through conscious work.

Freedom and the primary control are natural or inherent to the person. Limitation and poor use are acquired. To regain our right use of the primary control we stand free of the conditioned patterning. This requires awareness and intelligence of that patterning and its arising. The coordination basic to human movement and the characteristic patterning that overlays it are somatic (and kinaesthetically perceivable) and bodily (and outwardly observable).

To realize the natural state Alexander's general instruction is, at the initiation and through the progress of our actions, to *inhibit* or relax the habitual patterning and at the same time and all together *direct* or release oneself up from the place of support and outwards from the core while leaving the cycle of inspiration and expiration unrestricted. The manifestation of such freedom is obviously a complex and difficult undertaking, which is why it took Alexander years to work out for himself and why the guidance and facilitation of a teacher and an understanding of principles and practices are so important.

Our own conscious work is always required. Our first steps in that work are to walk through the looking glass and begin to pay attention.

A favourite story of mine begins with a Zen master entering a village and the villagers coming out to greet him. A spokesman steps forward and asks the master for instruction whereupon the master gestures for a writing tablet and writes the word, 'Attention'. The villager asks that the master offer clarification. Again the master gestures for the tablet and again writes 'Attention'. Perplexed and becoming impatient, the villager suggests that the master elucidate this important teaching and elaborate upon it. Once again the master motions for the tablet and this time writes 'Attention means attention.'

Attention to the somatic realm begins self-exploration and calls forth the vast intelligence of the human nervous system. Using the principles and practices of the Technique one applies intention as inhibition to relax the conditioned pattern and as direction to wish for and will the desired manner of action, which becomes more and more clear in feeling in the progress of practice.

Both inhibition and direction are mental gestures effective in the bodily realm. Though the line is fine neither inhibition nor direction involves physically doing anything. Inhibition is undoing or non-doing of the habit and direction is wishing and willing through means based on right principles. Alexander said that once you stop or inhibit the wrong 'thing' the right does itself. In the necessary process of our action direction helps that right along.

MOTOR CONCEPTS AND PERCEPTS

We lack sufficient conscious capacity to address the vast numbers of individual sensations and muscle actions pertaining to any moment of experience. In this method we work, rather, with motor concepts and percepts.

The senior motor concept is the primary control itself, which is not a sensation, muscle action, process or thing but the human manner of organizing movement in the actural dynamic, which can be accessed 'inwardly'. Other motor concepts we use are: up, down, out, away, forward, expansion, release, freedom, undoing and so on, which concepts have physical or motor referents: hence, *motor concepts*. Percepts, as somatic events accessible 'within', are, for instance, the skeleton (of which we have no direct sensation), the arms, legs, trunk, the body-as-a-whole, weight, directions, the cardinal lines (the central and peripheral axes of the body) and so forth. A percept is realized by the nervous system 'organizing' sensations. We can perceive the skeleton, for example, without any direct sensation of it by the nervous system's ability to integrate the sensory information from primarily the joint capsule receptors and muscle spindles and, in addition, the tendon and pressure receptors. Weight is a percept 'deduced' primarily from the tendon and pressure receptors. That aspect of the primary control that is proprioceptive – what Feldenkrais called the *primary image* – is a percept that involves the organization, correlation and interpretation of myriad sensory data.

Motor concepts and percepts act as a bridge between the mind and sensorimotor brain that we can work with consciously. In the progress of somatic learning, not only are our self-sensing and motor control refined directly through the manipulative processes, we also come to more accurately embody useful motor concepts and percepts enabling us to organize the system to better enact our intentions.

Using intention, you can make a fist, a doing. You can then not make the fist – an undoing. You can, via intention, open the hand, also a doing. Having opened the hand, you can, via intention, not do that anymore. Science cannot determine how the intention to make or unmake a fist and so on produces a neuromuscular response. Whatever intention, thought, intelligence, attention or any internal events are altogether is beyond the scope of this or any book.

Each of us in his or her *characteristic* manner is self-contracting and, in our response to events, we tend to contract in an *habitual* manner, the habitual and characteristic being closely related patterns. Inhibiting that conditioned patterning and then directing a new manner of action, the priorly free patterning, is the basic practice. We work largely with this core process. This singleness makes the Technique workable. The organization of movement as one thing accounts for the limitations of attention and simplifies work on oneself.

Getting a feel for the primary control is facilitated by what are called *positions of mechanical advantage*. These positions reveal the inherent relationships of the parts while putting the larger muscle groups in their mid-range where extraneous kinaesthetic 'noise' is minimized, allowing for better self-sensing and easier release. Semi-supine (see page 53) is the most passive of such positions. Sitting with one's hands upturned on one's thighs is also fairly passive. The so-called *monkey* position (see page 60) and its variations facilitate best organization while the body is in a tonic state.

A typical lesson involves sitting, standing, lying down, bending, reaching and walking, and, as we progress in practice, hands on the back of a chair and the whispered 'ah'. These are basic functions from which most other movements are elaborated. Similarly, the primary control as the foundation of all movement is the foreground of every lesson. A lesson in the Technique is, thus, self-study in the context of the basics of function, upon which we build a complex repertoire of functions in our daily lives. Working with foundation processes is one of the basic strategies in this work.

THE CAUSES OF PAIN

Where there are misalignment and shearing stresses, stiffness, compression and over-stimulation of pressure receptors, the contraction of stretched tissue and over-stimulation of tension receptors, ischemia or nerve impingement – the root of them all is, in general, chronic muscular contraction that is superfluous, inappropriate or parasitical to effective movement and responsive acture.

Pain may also be an effect of poor diet. A diet that includes an excess of foods that the body cannot adequately process and eliminate produces toxins that are shuffled off to tissues throughout the body. These poisons stimulate the free nerve endings scattered throughout the tissues, which stimulation is experienced as aches and pains. You may recall how you felt after a binge on alcohol or food. This is an acute example of excess of what otherwise may be chronic. The signs and symptoms of ageing may be the result of chronically inappropriate diet. Because the degenerative effects of such a diet are slow in their cumulative results, the day-to-day changes may not be observed, as per the Weber–Fechner principle, in the way they can be after a binge.

Few have a good idea of what represents a pure and purifying diet. This book is not a thesis on diet. I recommend study of such writers as Paavo Airola, Gary Null, Herbert Shelton, Paul C. Bragg, Arnold Ehret, Ann Wigmore, Victoria Boutenko and Adi Da Samraj for an intelligent understanding of a healthy diet. These teachers may seem like extremists compared to the average dietician but consideration of their ideas will convince one of their sanity and of the necessity to radically alter one's approach to food and food-taking.

Sometimes musculoskeletal or myofascial pain is chronic and continuous and no movement is possible without some pain. The approach in these instances is always to address it intelligently and seek to find the causes. With a first approximation to understanding, one can proceed, refining one's approximations as one learns.

Sometimes an issue can be addressed directly or locally. The Alexander Technique addresses the use of oneself as a whole. As a generalist approach to human function it accomplishes improvement in any specific problem through an improvement of the whole.

By organizing the core dynamic and thereby balancing the coordination of the whole structure, by minimizing muscular effort in the context of all activities, by reducing the action of muscles that are doing too much and bringing the appropriate degree of activity to muscles that are under-used, by thus freeing and expanding the body optimally and thereby indirectly undoing local and global patterns of undue contraction that are the causes of imbalances throughout the system, many pains are undermined at their source.

To practice in semi-supine, find a firm surface, a carpeted floor being about right. Lie down, bend the legs and bring the feet comfortably close to the buttocks. The feet should be far enough apart to enable the legs to balance with minimal effort, the knees neither falling apart nor together, but pointing to the ceiling; lay the back of the head on a pile of paperback books or something equally firm so that the front of the face is about flat. The books should not be in contact with the back of the neck. The height of the pile of books is different from person to person and will vary at different times for the same person. It depends on the length of the neck, the size of the head and the curvature of the spine. If you have too few books your head will tend to tilt backwards and it will be difficult to encourage release through the neck and back. If the pile is too high your chin will press down upon your throat and it will be difficult to encourage release through the neck and frontal line. Some people may be better aligned with no books at all. Place the hands by the sides or on the belly, stomach or chest. Make yourself comfortable. The low back may be resting on the floor.

Then scan the body, that is, sense yourself on the inside, even while knowing that your self-sensing is not completely trustworthy and needs refinement. Give your attention to the main parts of yourself: the head on the books, the neck between the head and trunk, the shoulder girdle and arms, the trunk, the front and back from the head to the pelvis, the bent legs and the feet on the floor. Attend to the fundamental directions: the primary line of the axial trunk from the pelvis through the head, and the cardinal lines of the limbs radiating out from the centre via the trunk. Wonder if there is anything you can let go so that you can settle more fully onto the floor.

Alexander described the primary control as a certain relativity of the head with the neck and of the head–neck relationship with the back and the rest of the body. With this image in mind try giving yourself directions: 'Let the neck be free, to let the head release forward and up (from the top of the neck), to let the back lengthen and widen, to let the arms release outwards via the shoulders, to let the legs release forward via the knees and away from each other via the hips, to let the axial line release out of the legs.' Give each consecutive order consciously and deliberately enough to connect the words and concepts to the corresponding parts and directions of the bodily self. Don't repeat the orders mechanically but rather as a conscious exercise of intention. Let the body open from the centre in all directions, as A.R. said, 'like a giant cauliflower'.

The head (in the actural dynamic) is poised on the top of the neck approximately between the ears at the atlanto-occipital joint. Releasing the neck frees the head–neck relationship. (Such release is accomplished by the same means as undoing a fist.) In that freedom, the head tends to revolve forward and up (in the body's frame of reference) relative to the neck because the head's centre of mass is forward and above its place of support on the atlas of the neck and the head is balanced via the rounded rockers of the occiput on the neck.

By freeing the neck, the back is free to lengthen and widen. To support the back's widening, you want the arms to release out of the top of the trunk and the legs to release out of the bottom of the trunk. You want the central axis, from the pelvis to the head, to release upwards from the legs at the hips following the head, and the body to release outwards from the centre via the widening of the trunk. Repeat this procedure of directing at random.

You may not feel that anything is happening but first you want to become aware of and intelligent about yourself as a whole and as a sum of parts and as a process of vectors. And part of what you are doing is learning the practice of Alexandrian thinking.

The body responds to intention and verbal thinking. If that response does not appear to be happening, understand that it may be happening and you are not yet sensitive enough to feel it; or it may not be happening but it will, because the brain-body does indeed respond to language and intention and may require time to work it out.

Anyway, you may notice the back resting more on the floor or feel it to be compressed. You may feel compression between the shoulders or in the neck or want to shift your position. You may begin to feel that the books are too high or that your arms or feet need adjusting. These signs indicate that your thinking is working and that the body is de-contracting or that you are becoming more aware through the practice. Try lying in semi-supine for twenty minutes at a trial. Repeat the procedure as often as you like.

Some of the value of semi-supine lies in the tactile information reflected via the floor, which, like a mirror, provides redundant information with which to compare the information from the self-senses and in the relaxation of the need to respond to gravity and the heightened sensory acuity thus afforded. An added mechanical benefit is that, in lying down for twenty minutes or so in the middle of the day, the intervertebral disks re-hydrate a little as the paraspinal musculature relaxes; the trunk thereby decompresses; and one feels lighter.

THE ACTURAL DYNAMIC

Because the head's centre of gravity is approximately between the temples, forward and above its place of support on the atlas vertebra of the spine, when the person is rightly organized in the actural dynamic, the back is always tending to lengthen upwards and the person to 'fall' forward. Because of this structural imbalance the body is always in a dynamic state of potency.

The response to gravity is centralized in the paraspinal muscles of the back and generalized in the extensor musculature altogether. A muscle is most efficient when it is maximally released and has the most available contractibility. When the extensor musculature is maximally released in the practice of the Technique the response to gravity is efficient and easy and there is a consequent lightness in the quality of action and feeling.

The support offered by the skeleton as a compression structure is one of the ways that effort in the response to gravity is minimized and the feeling of lightness optimized. (A brick wall is a simple compression structure.) The myofascial network in conjunction with the skeleton, which together function as a complex tensegrity structure, plays a greater supportive role in the gravitational response. (A sailing ship is a simple tensegrity structure where the mast is held upright, the spars balanced and supported and the sail supported and suspended by the mechanical tension of the stays. In simplistic terms, from the axial 'mast' that is the upright human body, erected via the 'stays' of the extensor system, is suspended the 'spar' that is the shoulder girdle, from which is suspended the 'sail' that is the ribcage, the 'stays' from which balance the 'spar' that is the pelvic girdle.) The spine with its spongy disks, the watery nature of the body and the arches of the feet work all together as a compression spring. There are other mechanical properties, such as hydraulics, in terms of air and water pressure within the body, that serve the gravitational response. Stretch reflexes, equilibrium reactions, postural reflexes, righting reflexes and positive support reactions also contribute to the gravitational response.

The response to gravity is reflexive. Freedom of the body must be conscious if it isn't spontaneous because our reactions to stressors tend to be unconscious and effective and we must exert a senior force to counter them.

We are as supported in our radical uprightness by the reflex response to gravity 'inside us' as is a fish by the water 'outside it'. There is no weight in the body; it is under our feet. Limitations imposed by function and structure do not in principle limit our use. We are not merely structures and functions but psychophysical beings wherein our mental processes inform and shape our function and structure. No matter what is imposed on us we can always pay attention and think intelligently and thus have access to freedom in action. Hence, Alexander's hyperbolic claim that his best student was a hunchbacked elderly lady.

As you come to some clarity in semi-supine, you might try sitting with the hands on the lap. Again you want a firm support as the firmness of the seat gives clearer information of the place of contact and offers better support for the back than a soft surface. Follow the same mental procedures of directing so that it is a mentally active sitting.

You may try leaning forward and backwards from the sitting bones, intending that the trunk be integrated, supple and buoyant, neither rigid nor flaccid. The trunk should move from the 'joint' of the sitting bones with the chair. The legs should be free at the hips, released forward from the back and away from each other, to allow the back to move, so that the knees move freely forward and backward with the forward and backward leaning of the trunk.

THE HIP JOINTS, THE MOVEMENT OF THE PELVIS AND GROUNDING

The hip joints are pivotal to the body in action. Their function is often compromised in people today because of a sedentary lifestyle, the ergonomics of furniture and the close association between the hip joints and the functions of sex and excretion, which may be complicated. By the time a person reaches adulthood, the immobility of the pelvis and hips can be of a structural nature where functional work is inadequate to address the myofascial restrictions. There are normally twenty-six muscles and several ligaments that cross each hip joint, many of which may be limited in their mobility and malleability. A possible solution is a progressive program of yoga.

One virtue of a yoga practice is that ordinary activities do not generally engage the connective tissue beyond a narrow range. Thus, over time, the myofascial network can become dense and inflexible. Yoga extends this subnormal range and keeps the body limber and mobile. The hip joints are ball-and-socket joints that potentially allow for a range of movement through more than a hemisphere. A graduated yoga regimen that works towards this range while seeking to achieve a balanced flexibility throughout the structure is a good idea.

In working with freeing the hips and the consequent greater awareness of the movement of the pelvis and its connection to the legs a person feels better supported and functionally grounded.

Challenging yourself in monkey is a big next step once you have achieved some competency in semi-supine and sitting. The directions are the same. In the beginning, leave the arms relaxed. With practice, you may try raising them in a gesture of beholding. You can increase the challenge of the position by deepening the bending of the knees or changing the angle of the back.

MORE ON GIVING DIRECTIONS

The basic directions given by Alexander for organizing the primary control are: 'Let the neck be free, to let the head go forward and up, to let the back lengthen and widen, to let the legs go forward and away, to let the shoulders release apart – all at once, one after another.'

Let us examine these directions in further detail in our first approach to learning the Technique for ourselves.

'Let the neck be free.' Patrick MacDonald once remarked that he had observed many beginning students going through all sorts of contortions in the belief that they were freeing the neck where they were often producing more stiffening. Letting the neck be free is rather a not-doing, thereby undoing whatever one is habitually doing with the neck, which is always some stiffening or contracting. Letting the neck be free is of the same nature as letting go a fist.

'(To) let the head go forward and up.' The head's centre of mass is between the temples and the head's place of support, on the top of the cervical spine, between the ears on the atlas vertebra. The bottom of the skull is shaped like the rockers of a rocking chair. The head is thus always already tending to revolve forward and up from its place of support. The musculature of the trunk and neck, when rightly released, allows the head to do that. Thus, directing the head to go forward and up is about letting it do what it will naturally do if it is free to do so.

'(To) let the back lengthen and widen.' Alexander likened the lengthening and widening of the back to the smoothing of a crumpled sheet of paper, which will, in that smoothing, expand in its two dimensions. When the neck and head are free, the back is no longer compressed from above and will spontaneously release in its dimensions of length and (with the release of the arms and legs) of width if it is allowed to do so. Thus directing the back is, like the other directions, a matter of allowing and intending the inherent freedom of the core dynamic.

'(To) let the legs release forward and away.' The femurs are shaped like canes that angle laterally from the pelvis at the hip joint and then take a sharp bend straight to the knees. The legs' natural directions therefore are away from each other at the hips via the 'handle of the cane' and, in the semi-supine, seated and monkey positions (and not so obviously in standing) forward from the pelvis. So directing the legs has them do what they will spontaneously do if allowed to do so.

'(To) let the shoulders release up and away.' The shoulder girdle, the first link of the arms, is shaped rather like two wishbones pointing laterally from the top of the ribcage. It is 'lifted' from the ribcage and suspended from the neck and head via the 'stays' of the scalene, sternocleidomastoid, trapezius, levator scapulae and other muscles and ligaments. Thus the natural direction of the shoulders is up and away from the ribcage.

'All at once one after another' – because the mechanism is a sequentially organized functional integrity.

As Alexander remarked, what we are doing in this work is exactly what is happening in Nature when conditions are right, only we are learning to do it consciously. If you examine the human form when all the muscles are in a state of maximal release as in an untrained astronaut in zero gravity these relationships and directions are manifest.

Positions of mechanical advantage provide a progressive way to 'locate' the primary control, which can allow you to randomly address your coordination and functioning during the day. You may start to consider yourself in a new way and regain a sense of awareness and control that transforms your relationship with your body.

It may be apparent to you that monkey with the hands in a gesture of beholding is the ready position for boxing, wrestling and the martial arts and, in its lunge variation, for a foot race.

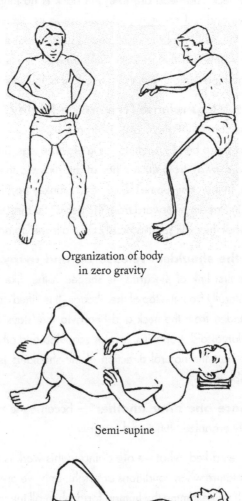

Organization of body
in zero gravity

Semi-supine

Semi-supine on a roller

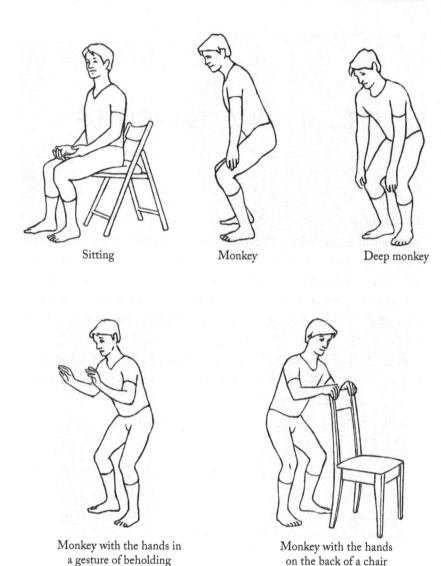

Sitting   Monkey   Deep monkey

Monkey with the hands in
a gesture of beholding

Monkey with the hands
on the back of a chair

(The limitation of a picture as a communication of what the practice is in the context of the Alexander Technique or any somatic work is that a picture cannot illustrate the dynamic nature of the pose or movement or the workings of the mind applied to the sensorimotor processes or the subject's idiosyncratic structure.)

ORGANIZING PRINCIPLES

According to esoteric tradition the individual is an integrated hierarchical psychophysical process whose essence is the 'attention' (that is the root function of the causal body) upon which depends the senior subordinate function of intelligence whose central instruments are the faculties of observation and intention. Thinking, emotional feeling, sensing and acting follow from these. The Alexander Technique uses the functions of the 'attention' (that is interested observation), intelligence, intention and thinking to elicit improvements in the subordinate functions of sensing, acting and, rather indirectly, emotion.

All the principles are interwoven and interactive.

USE

Alexander chose the term 'use' to describe something about how a person thinks or exercises the mind in the context of sensorimotor functioning; how a person senses and organizes movement; and the how of the organization itself. Alexander named his most succinct book *The Use of the Self.* He called an earlier work *Constructive Conscious Control of the Individual* which meant the same.

Use is the measure of present-time conscious intelligence and freedom brought to the sensorimotor process. You might say that the 'physical effect' of our use is our *self-organization.*

We can harmonize the manner we carry out any action and we can also refine the quality of intelligence we bring to sensorimotor function. Improving sensorimotor reliability is accomplished in the Technique primarily by the use of the mind as it is brought to bear upon our organization. The Alexander Technique is also of course manipulative. That, in conjunction with pertinent instruction, Alexander discovered to be the most effective means whereby he could facilitate somatic learning. But manipulation is subordinate in principle to the use of the mind. Thomas Hanna said that 'the body is an artifact of the soma', that is, how we function depends upon what we are doing on the 'inside' – our awareness, our intelligence, our intention and choices, our thinking, our feeling and our self-sensing.

Use affects functioning and is prior and primary to functioning. It is also true that our functioning affects our use but the relationship is not equal. Everyone has noticed that the flu makes one's thinking less clear. The repetition of destructive habits undermines the quality of life. If the wheels of the caboose are broken and the axles twisted, the whole train is going to run inefficiently. However, if the engine is not working the train is not going to move at all.

ATTENTION (INTERESTED OBSERVATION)

For a moment, give your attention to your left hand. What you just did on the inside can't be seen or measured but, whatever it was, that is attention or interested observation. The first 'object' of one's attention in this work is the primary control, the means whereby of action, accessed inwardly. As one moves into or through an action attention is coupled with the step-by-step organization of the action.

Paying attention to the manner of movement is not easy. The practice obviously involves the body with which some of us are out of touch. As inheritors of cultures founded on the exoteric religious and typical esoteric spiritual views that eschew the body and on the emotional concomitants of that attitude, we may have learned to suppress, be embarrassed about or even be dismissive of bodily life or to react against this negative disposition and exploit our bodily possibilities, or both. A wrong view may stem from schooling where we may have learned to disregard our functional needs in favour of intellectual or social gains. For some, there has been physical neglect or sexual or physical abuse.

Such issues are not directly addressed in the Technique. The Technique seeks to reinforce the understanding that 'I am the body' and not inside, outside, separate from or other than it.

Even when the body is clearly giving pain signals it may be ignored. Having pain can be a reason for not paying attention to it. Pain is sensory information often indicating faulty patterns of action.

Our manner of movement is difficult to attend to because we are not often merely attentive to the present moment of action. We tend to be oriented to the goal of our actions. Even a dancer or yogi who may do very complex movements is not typically merely present to his or her movements but often performs such movements in order to approximate a form projected from outside the self.

The primary control involves the core musculature of the body, what Feldenkrais called 'the idiot within'. In general, we do not move these areas competently and are rarely aware of them. Interestingly, we do not have much neurophysiological access to these parts. The majority of the sensorimotor cortex is apportioned to the hands, lips, tongue and vocal apparatus and only about a quarter of that cortex to the rest of the body. Remarkably there is as much of the cortex devoted to the use of the thumb as the entire trunk and legs. Thus, sensing and controlling those parts that comprise the primary control is simply difficult.

INTELLIGENCE

Human intelligence expresses itself as play, exploration, intuition, interest, reason, consideration, reflection, investigation, creativity, study, work, discrimination, insight, learning, understanding, knowing and so on.

Knowledge of principles is valuable to quicken sensorimotor competence. Intelligence must inform practice on an ongoing basis in the form of continued self-exploration and consideration of principles. Whatever we can know about the functioning of the body as a physical mechanism can serve that functioning, sometimes in obvious ways. If, as a member of the Flat Earth Society, you newly discover that the world is round you are immediately free of the fear of falling off the edge of the earth and you might feel interested in exploring. Similarly, when you know something about the way the body works, that knowledge informs the way you function. This is the essence of 'body-mapping', a practice devised and developed by the American Alexander teacher, Barbara Conable.

Percepts and motor concepts act as the cognitive bridge between intelligence and the sensorimotor processes. It is their simplicity and familiarity that make the Technique simple in principle: up, down, out, away, forward, expansion, release, freedom, undoing, the skeleton, arms, legs, the trunk, the body-as-a-whole, weight, the cardinal lines and so on. The better the grasp and embodiment of these concepts and percepts, the truer self-sensing and motor function become.

Conscious intelligence rides on the self-organizing capability of the nervous system, which in the human case is immense. Any kind of work or play that calls for our attention calls forth the nervous system's response. The line between the conscious and unconscious is vague and we move back and forth between them.

After Alexander resolved his own troubles and others became interested in how he had done it he first instructed people verbally. He soon discovered that instructing them manually – not fixing them, but rather informing and facilitating their sensorimotor intelligence by giving them new experiences of themselves – was far more effective. This discovery is original to the Technique.

While chiropractors, massage therapists, physiotherapists and such use their hands to change people, it is only teachers of the Alexander Technique – and, more recently, other somatic educators – who are working with their student's capacity for sensorimotor learning. Understanding this difference between the modalities of medical treatment and of somatic education may necessitate a paradigm shift on the part of the individual seeking self-improvement through these methods. A teacher of the Technique may appear to palpate tissue and move various parts of the body as a massage therapist or physiotherapist may do. But the purposes are fundamentally different. The Alexander teacher is seeking to understand how the person is organizing him- or herself in terms of movement and the response to gravity and to understand how and what he or she is thinking and sensing in terms of mechanics and function in general. A therapist generally does not have such ideas in mind because such a therapist does not generally conceive of him- or herself as working with present-time sensorimotor intelligence and the ability to learn.

Alexander teachers use their bodies as sensory mechanisms. The teacher is sensing via his or her hands the pupil's coordination holistically, taking in the whole pupil via the primary control, the manner of action.

While it is true that the sensorimotor process cannot be directly manipulated by another, the Alexander teacher, by skilful interventions, may call forth the response of the pupil's nervous system and, it is hoped, his interest. Indeed, without the evocation of interest, the person cannot begin to be an agent in his or her own improvement.

THE PRIMARY CONTROL

The primary control is the senior organizing function of movement, perceivable inwardly and outwardly, its parts to be organized 'all at once, one after another'. This is so because what we are doing in this work is exactly what happens in Nature when conditions are right, only we are doing it consciously.

When a train engine moves, the passenger cars, the flat cars, the cargo cars and the caboose all move at exactly the same time. Without the engine moving first, nothing else can follow. In conjunction with the human body's uniquely high centre of gravity the freedom of the primary control facilitates optimal conditions for movement, making the structure functionally weightless.

Feldenkrais demonstrated that the movement of the eyes organizes the movement of the body. To differentiate Feldenkrais' from Alexander's view and see how they are both true, understand that the use of the eyes 'informs' movement where the primary control 'forms' movement: you can turn your eyes to, say, follow the passage of a car and not turn your head with the eyes and, as long as you keep the body releasing and directed up from the support and outwards from the centre, it is a good movement.

As we learn to move well we become more sensitive to ourselves and, as we reduce the distracting kinaesthetic noise of our own habits, to others – and we feel better. This sensitivity to oneself and thence to others is the essence of the teacher's craft because his sensory system has attention and energy freed from binding patterning.

SENSORIMOTOR UNRELIABILITY

Alexander found that he literally did not know what he was doing in terms of the biomechanical functions. This is the paradox of unconsciousness. Later he discovered that this problem is endemic. Any unresolved pain, conflict or difficulty in life brings the fact and meaning of unconsciousness to one's attention.

When a person suffers from a functional or structural problem he or she must be unaware in terms of sensorimotor function, otherwise he would already not be doing the 'thing' that is harmful or problematic. And so, he has to learn to sense again how he is doing what he is doing.

There are real causes for our faulty patterns of functioning. But whatever was in the past it is only the present functioning that can be addressed and that is a combined sensory and motor matter.

There is a remarkable story in *Constructive Conscious Control of the Individual* (Alexander 2004), which illustrates this point vividly: 'A little girl who had been unable to walk properly for some years was brought to me for a diagnosis of the defects in the use of the psychophysical mechanisms which were responsible for her more or less crippled state. When this had been done a request was made that a demonstration be given to those present of the manipulative side of the work (the child, the subject to be manipulated) so that certain readjustments and co-ordinations might be temporarily secured, thus showing, in keeping with the diagnosis, the possibilities of re-education on a general basis in a case of this kind. The demonstration was successful from this point of view. For the time being the child's body was comparably straightened out, that is, without the extreme twists and distortions that had been so noticeable when she came into the room. When this was done, the little girl looked across at her mother and said to her in an indescribable tone, "Oh! Mommy, he's pulled me all out of shape!'"

This girl's experience is not uncommon during lessons. Once in my own training my teacher was working with me in standing and, with one of his hands on my back, asked, 'Which way are you leaning?' I thought for a moment, came to a firm conclusion, and replied, 'Forward.' He removed his hand and I staggered backwards.

Many similar experiences can be described during lessons. Pupils will feel in the lesson as though they are standing like an ape or that the butt is sticking out or that they are leaning forward or backward. In the typical case, they will be quite wrong. They will be clearly more upright than they were. More often pupils will say they feel more relaxed, taller and broader, and they will be quite right. How can both perceptions be true?

When a person organizes him- or herself in a characteristic manner – say, always raising the shoulders – then, when the shoulders are floating on the ribcage, the person will almost inevitably feel that they are 'down', 'rounded' or 'collapsed' or some such misperception of the new sensations. Many examples could be described of changes in a person's self-organization and the consequent self-perception. The unfamiliar feelings, both 'good' and 'bad', that accompany the new organization are relatively accurate and, so, relatively inaccurate and are therefore not reliable, and they are secondary to the changes in self-organization.

Chronic pains are the tip of the iceberg of sensorimotor unreliability. When a person has been using him- or herself poorly for an extended period of time or, as a result of a recent trauma, for a short period of time, pain may result. But the removal of pain, which often accompanies early work in the Technique, rarely represents a resolution of causes but more often only the undoing of gross misuse. When someone comes for lessons with chronic or recurrent pain as the presenting symptom, many lessons are required to master the deep-seated patterns of misuse that are the source of the pain and limitation. If a person ends lessons before a virtuous spiral of improvement is initiated and an individual practice established it is not unlikely that the symptoms will recur or new symptoms arise.

SELF-CORRECTION

Walter Carrington once quipped that once you become a student of the Technique, from then on, you know only when you are going wrong. Any direct effort to correct oneself, however, will tend to be ineffective. Rather, what is right will, as Alexander said, do itself once the wrong is inhibited and the right 'relocated'.

Direction should not be made in the mood and mode of self-correction, what Alexander called 'end-gaining'. The intention to directly correct oneself inevitably manifests partially and becomes, as John Dewey remarked, 'a different kind of badly'. To that 'correction' the whole system will by its nature globally adapt, exacerbating the 'badly'. Awareness and intelligence and the impulse to freedom allow for self-correction to emerge spontaneously via learning. Inhibition informed by our growing intelligence of the primary control is the means to this end. We become more and more able to whole-bodily feel towards what is free and effective as a hand feels into a glove. But that more reliable feeling cannot be taken for granted. As Alexander remarked towards the end of his life, he continued to do the work, otherwise he would go wrong.

SELF-CONTRACTION

Each of us tends to be always active as a unique complex bodily pattern that defines the personality. Moshe Feldenkrais and Thomas Hanna identified root patterns of effort, anxiety and protection. I add the pattern of collapse. When a person counters such collapse with what is a necessary effort to 'hold himself up' he adopts a personal compensating global pattern to accomplish this. Even when he thus efforts to 'holds himself up', the feel of such a person is always 'down' because the collapse is not undone in the effort, merely covered. In his book, *Emotional Anatomy*, Stanley Keleman claims to describe a pantheon of habituated patterns that bodily express emotional character. Charles Darwin and Konrad Lorenz identified a collection of fundamental emotions that are bodily expressed in animals and man and may become habituated.

All such conditioned patterning is parasitical to the buoyant response to gravity that is native to us and can be seen beautifully demonstrated in undamaged children. This buoyant anti-gravity response can be rediscovered through conscious work. It is not that a person can or should always be straight and tall. On the contrary, any number of possible expressions should be available to a person. It is the chronic, unconscious, compulsive or stereotyped nature of such patterning that is their liability.

Still, it may be worth considering if emotional reaction patterns could be undermined by not using the body in the way that expresses those patterns. This may be the basis of Ida Rolf's contention that the process of change is irrelevant, that what matters is the changed state that does not afford the expression of what she called neurotic patterns.

The Technique does not work directly with emotional, psychological or character strategies at the root of any individual's patterning. Nor does it work with any causative factors in the past. It works with the present 'cause', which the individual manifests as reduced self-awareness and understanding of his own process, reduced facility to connect his intention to action and deficient self-organization. With improving use, the subjective factors that may be correlated with the patterns of limitation are either revealed indirectly and so made available to address by other means or obviated through being deprived of their means of expression.

Remarkably, the stress response, as Hans Selye (1978) identified it in his seminal research, not only involves a 'general adaptation syndrome' of endocrine responses but a global neuromuscular reflex reaction pattern wherein every muscle of the body increases in tone, resulting in a pattern of contraction in towards the centre and, because of our generally upright functioning in the actural dynamic, down in the direction of gravity along the axial line. Practice of the Technique thus effectively undermines the sensorimotor manifestations of the stress response and, in that process, you may more often find a spirit of lightness and ease in everyday life.

HOLISM

Alexander discovered through self-study that we are a hierarchically integrated complex functional system. The understanding of the holistic organization of movement as the present-time shaping of action allows for a unique means of self-improvement that can be practiced here in the body and now in movement. The organization of the whole body in action becomes more and more available to 'conscious control' as a person progresses in mastery of the method and of him- or herself as a functional integrity.

The primary control can be apprehended as a gestalt. This notion is validated by neurophysiological research that indicates that the brain perceives and actualizes what are called 'mass movements': from the point of view of the soma the musculoskeletal network is one thing that is organized moment to moment in different patterns according to the requirements of the action.

Whether the movement is reaching with the arms, thrusting with the legs, turning the head or lunging with the trunk, whatever action is performed, it is always done with all of oneself with more or less of each part involved in the action of the whole.

INTENTION

Intention in the forms of inhibition and direction is the means whereby intelligence is enacted. In the beginning, inhibition takes the form of stopping or relinquishing the habitual response to an inner or outer stimulus to act. In an Alexander lesson, the stimuli are reduced to the intention to sit, stand, bend and so on, so that the practice of 'refusing to respond habitually' to a stimulus can be established more easily than it can be in a complex action. Then inhibition takes the form of release and resolution of the individual pattern of self-contracting, which is an interference with best organization.

Direction first takes the release of inhibition further and, in that sense, inhibition and direction are like two sides of a single coin. Then direction takes the form of 'sending' messages to the motor system to enact the action pattern desired.

The nervous system or the unconscious mind knows where everything in the body is and how it works. It heals our wounds, puts together all our complex movements according to our will and so forth. The conscious process is to bypass our obstructive habits through the exercise of worded intentions and direct the nervous system to rightly organize the physical mechanism.

Verbal intentions are effective because the body responds to the force and meaning of language. Our grasp of any word, motor concept or percept becomes more refined as we become more sensitive to our physical selves. Words have value relative to the sensorimotor intelligence attached to them. Children in their learning, but also anyone suffering sensorimotor unreliability, cannot do the things exactly as they are told. As one reacquaints oneself with the body there comes a growing ability to move effectively. All learning takes time. Some trial and error is inevitable. Good coordination is not a spontaneous matter but a developmental and educational one.

The thought of an action is sufficient to innervate the muscles that habitually perform it. Thus, the habitual action founded on that thought must be inhibited and a new means whereby that intended action can be learned. You cannot change what you don't know you're doing. Proportional to your awareness and intelligence is your capacity to inhibit and direct. In order to increase your awareness or ability to sense yourself, use of the musculature is useful, because of the cybernetic-like feedback relationship between movement and self-sensing. The simple movements used in an Alexander lesson provide a basic range of sensations to stimulate awareness from which further learning can be generalized. Awareness Through Movement is also helpful in this regard.

Such slow designed movement sequences draw attention to parts presently unavailable to awareness and can then serve the integration of those parts. In the Alexander Technique, tonic contraction of major muscle groups is stimulated through monkey and its variations. These tonic positions can stimulate awareness to areas and patterns presently inaccessible. In some cases, assisted pandiculation – made an explicit handling strategy in Thomas Hanna's work – which is an assisted strong measured contraction in the context of mass movements followed by a slow controlled release of that contraction – is helpful to wake up these areas. Such pandiculations work at the neurophysiological level similarly to the strong tonic contractions required for a deep monkey stimulating a great amount of afferent information to the sensory cortex and thus directly informing motor function. They use the Weber–Fechner principle to 'speak more loudly' than the noise of contraction patterns.

THE FOUR IMAGINARY CENTRES

Without an adequate response to gravity in which human movement takes place movement lacks a right ground. No matter how flexible a person or how strong or how relaxed, if he or she does not competently counter the constant force of gravity, gravity wins. This is the basis for the Technique's constant address to the primary control of action and the reason why variety of movement plays a secondary role in an Alexander lesson. A typical lesson involves sitting, standing, bending, reaching, walking and lying down, basic actions upon which most other actions can be built. All of these simple actions are mini-laboratories for studying oneself in the context of one's way of movement in gravity.

The nature of the response to gravity is determined by the relationship of the human physical mechanism to the planet where the centre of gravity of that relationship is essentially at the earth's centre. This fact makes this centre the greater organizing factor in human function and creates the primary direction 'up'.

The vital centre of the mechanism and the centre of gravity of the body in movement creates the secondary directions 'out'.

The centre of mass of the head, located approximately between the temples, is forward and above its place of support on top of the neck. Thus, the head is always tending forward and up off the top of the spine. The earth determines acture or the response to gravity. The vital centre determines movement. The leading of the head – or third centre – defines the direction of movement.

Limitations in the response to gravity are constant and characteristic; in movement, recurrent and habitual.

The fourth 'centre' is the axis of the body. All contracting, whether on one side of this line or in front or in back of it or around it, requires an antagonistic co-contraction somewhere to maintain balance in the actural dynamic. For example, pulling down in the front requires a compensating pulling down somewhere in the back for balance. Contraction on one side necessitates contraction somewhere on the other. A rotational contraction requires a twist elsewhere. Compression is always the effect of such co-contraction.

THE FRONTAL LINE

The frontal line described in esoteric traditions as the circuit of descending life-energy, which turns about at the bodily base and ascends via the spinal line, tends to be obstructed, according to Adi Da Samraj, via the 'vital shock' that is the reaction to apparently separate, apparently vulnerable, born existence. This energetic/emotional blockage manifests as the sense of separation from the Source of Life, doubt, suppression of life-energy and of love, anger, sorrow and fear, and as contraction of the frontal musculature, with its focal point in the vital centre. This is, I believe, a reason for the focus in the martial arts, which are psychophysical disciplines of the frontal line, on the opening and strengthening of and 'grounding' in the vital centre.

Much of the frontal musculature serves assimilation, elimination, respiration, perception, expression and communication, is only minimally involved in motor and anti-gravity functions, and ordinarily needs to be essentially relaxed. Frontal line contraction is evident in strained facial expressions, constriction of the voice, pulling down or collapse of the chest, deficient breathing, hyper-tonicity of the abdominal wall, retraction of the pelvis and tightening of the pelvic floor and navel, the gripping of the hip joints and so forth and counteractions to those patterns. In order to resolve such issues so that the back can properly lengthen, the release of the frontal line should happen together with the freeing of the other elements basic to the primary control. In the directions used in orthodox practice, this is not directly addressed. Making this address explicit within the framework of directing may be helpful for some.

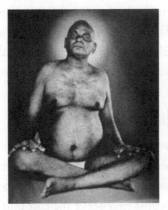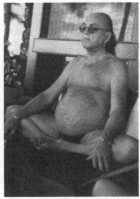

The open frontal line is here manifest in Swami Nityananda, the source guru of the Siddha yoga tradition, and in Adi Da Samraj, the source guru of Adidam.

TENSEGRITY

It requires an effort of will to fall over and none to stand. The reflexive response to gravity establishes our uprightness and the mechanism then functions in the actural dynamic essentially as a tensegrity structure. Monkey with the arms in a gesture of beholding or with hands on the back of a chair is the archetype of all action in the actural dynamic and epitomizes the system as a tensegrity structure. By working with cantilever-like effects, the monkey position takes the head forward and up from the top of the spine, lengthening the back from the top, while the weight of the pelvis cantilevering over the hip joints draws the back down, lengthening the spine from the bottom, the elastic tissue of the back functioning thus as a stay. The knees release forward while the back is directed back and the heels released into the floor, the extensor myofascia of the legs functioning again as stays. The shoulders and arms as a whole are released in opposite directions from each other and from the back while the weight of the arms, which takes them forward and down, opposes the directing of the back and the arms as an extension of the back up and back. All this serves to lengthen and widen the back, stimulating appropriate tone as in the tension of a stay. The action of the extensor system of the back relaxes the frontal musculature and the tilting forward of the trunk further relaxes the frontal musculature and tones the back.

HABIT, LEARNING AND FREEDOM

Self-contracted patterns have myriad causes and may become habitual if not resolved by alternative action. The Technique's purpose is to free the individual from habitual action and reaction. A lesson initiates this process in simple activities. One begins to observe the compulsiveness or habit of one's reaction in simple movements and then brings to bear upon that compulsiveness attention, intelligence and intention – what Dewey called 'thinking in activity' – and thereby learns a new manner of action.

As one becomes more and more free of negative habits, one has more energy and attention available for the refinement of ability. Because these newly acquired habits have been learned consciously, they can be accessed at will and built upon, re-organized or relinquished. There is a movement to and from conscious and unconscious control.

Lessons

A FIRST POSSIBLE LESSON

'The Alexander Technique is a practice of applying the mind to the mechanics of movement and the sensorimotor process altogether. By mind, I mean the mental faculties of attention, intelligence and intention.

'By attention, I mean, can you pay attention to your left knee right now? Now, I don't know what you did. A scientist can't come into the room and measure some event that occurred in the physical universe. It's a mental event.

'When we begin to pay attention to the body we can apply our intelligence to it. By intelligence, I mean your capacity to think (intelligently, of course), reason, consider, explore, work creatively, play, intuit, know, learn, understand, guess, wonder and so on. All these are activities of intelligence and we use them here because, if we are using our intelligence, we can make positive changes.

'By intention I mean this: make a fist; now, open the hand. Make a fist again. Now, instead of opening the hand, just stop making the fist.

'Right.

'So you understand the difference. The first is a doing – making a fist or opening the hand. The second is an undoing. No one knows what intention is or how it accomplishes either, but it obviously does, so we use it in the Technique to effect the changes that are release and attuning of the mechanism, release of the unnatural patterns and attuning to or relocation of the natural pattern.

'It was Alexander's observation that each of us, in his or her own unique way, is doing something at all times and in all activities, doing in the sense of making a fist of all of ourselves – and this doing is observable and recognizable. For instance, you can recognize a friend at a distance because of a characteristic complex global patterning.

'So the first means we use in the Technique is the inhibition and resolution of this overlay of pattern. The second means we use is the evocation of and attuning to the underlying natural pattern, which Alexander discovered and called the primary control. The primary control is the unique natural human manner of organizing movement in the context of the human response to gravity.

'If you think of a snake slithering along the floor here, it doesn't matter if the snake is green, brown, black, striped, diamond-backed, whatever – as soon as you see that movement, you recognize a snake. Similarly, you have probably seen a wildlife program set in Africa. It doesn't matter if the creature you are looking at is a lion, panther, cheetah or leopard, as soon as you see that movement, you recognize feline movement and not canine movement. Or you will have seen one of those little creatures running across the street here in Toronto. Again, it doesn't matter if the animal is black or grey or brown – as soon as you see that movement, you recognize a squirrel and can distinguish it from a rat.

'The primary control is the human manner of organizing movement. And it is as recognizable as that of a snake, a squirrel or a cat. If John Candy is dressed in an ape suit standing beside a real ape, as soon as one of them moves, you know which is the ape and which, the man. The way that humans organize movement, what Alexander called the primary control, is immediately recognizable. It involves the dynamics and coordination of relationship of the head with the neck and of the head–neck relationship with the back and, via the centre, with the rest of the body and via the pelvis and legs, with the ground.

'To organize our movement well, we must organize the primary control well because it is the core dynamic of our movement to which we can pay attention, consider intelligently, and, via the mind's interaction with the mechanism, free and control.

'The primary control is native to the mechanism. While we are seeking right control of the mechanism, because the primary control is natural, what we are really seeking is to free ourselves of the patterns with which we have overlaid or obstructed the inherent pattern so that the inherent pattern can manifest.

'In the lesson, we are not working with movement *per se*, but rather *in* movement *with* the organization of movement. The organization of movement is subtle. In a lesson then, we generally work with simple movements, so that we are not distracted from the subtleties of the primary control by complex movements.

'So, standing here in front of the stool as though to sit, you want to begin to give your attention to yourself and consider the whole thing.

'The primary control is not a thing. It's not the body. It's not a process. It's not even the process of upright movement. Rather, it is a way, the human manner of action. It is the dynamic organization of upright movement in the actural dynamic. And that organization is like a train's. If you think of a train, with the cars all linked up, when the engine moves, the passenger cars, the flat cars, the cargo cars and the caboose all move at exactly the same time. Like a train, our manner of movement is sequential, instant and integrated. Your access to that organization is through attention, intelligence and intention. My access to it is with my hands and eyes and words.

'Alexander found that to use ourselves well, our address must be sequential, instant and all together, that is, all at once, one part after another, and in an integrated way.

'The first link in the primary control is the head–neck relationship. The first thing to free, then, is the head–neck relationship so that the rest of the mechanism can freely follow. Now, you free the head–neck relationship the same way as you free the fist – by an intention to undo.

'Alexander's instruction was to free the neck. The neck connects the head and back. The musculature of the neck and its relationship to the head are very similar to the musculature of the hand and its relationship, say, to a ball it is holding. Just as you release the fingers' hold circling the ball, so you release the neck, front, back and sides, and its hold on the head, the muscles of the neck extending up and around the head like the fingers of the hand.

'So freeing the neck allows the neck to lengthen, the head to release from the neck, which initiates the freedom of the back. Because the centre of mass of the head is forward and above its base of support on the top of the neck, when you free the neck, the head will tend to revolve forward and up from the top of neck.

'So, you find that you cannot do that so easily. Not to worry. Your problems have only begun.

'Just kidding.

'So, you find that accessing the neck and the head–neck relationship is not as easy as accessing the hand.

'Even though you may feel nothing, you should know that the musculature of the head-neck region bears the same relationship to your understanding as the musculature of the hand, and so what we want to do here in the beginning is exercise the mind anyway for the mere sake of learning the method of Alexandrian thinking.

'At the same time as you begin to free the head–neck relationship, you want to free the back. Where the neck is one-dimensional and when you free it, it will tend to lengthen, the back is two-dimensional and when you free it, it will tend to both lengthen and widen.

'We lack much neurological access to the back. But we must address the back anyway as the head-neck-back dynamic is key to organizing our action in an effortless way.

'Following these primary directions relative to freeing the head-neck-back dynamic, we want to direct the legs to release forward from the back or pelvis and away from each other – that is, out of the centre altogether – and the shoulders, up and away from each other – again, out of the centre.

'When we have all this thinking going, only then are we ready to take action – to, say, sit down.

'But don't sit down.

'Continue thinking your directions relative to freeing the neck, releasing the head forward and up from the top of the spine, allowing the back to lengthen and widen, the shoulders to release apart and the legs to release forward and away. And then consider how to sit down while keeping all those directions going.

'Ideally every movement would be done in the context of releasing the body up from its place of support and out of the centre. Sitting down then is not about going down but about folding at the hips, knees and ankle joints – while going up and out in the context of the primary control – and you find yourself on the chair.

'Similarly, to stand up, you get your thinking going as before and then you simply go with the forward momentum of hinging forward on the sitting bones without disorganizing the trunk and, as you bring your centre of gravity over the feet, you follow your head into standing. The movement is virtually effortless.

'It may not feel right. It probably won't feel familiar.

'The movements here are unimportant. It is the manner of organizing the movements that is important. On the other hand, sitting and standing are fundamental human activities and their right organization informs many other daily movements.

'So then, let's come back to sitting, coordinating the primary control as before, as Alexander said, all at once, one after another.

'OK.

'Now let me tell you about the arm. Both developmentally and functionally, the shoulder girdle – the clavicle and scapula – is part of the arm. So the arm doesn't start at the shoulder joint but rather comes off the ribcage via its first link, the shoulder girdle.

'When I pick up your arm like this by your hand, I am looking to feel the arm's connection to and freedom from the ribcage – as a link in a chain is both free of and connected to the next link.

'At the same time, the whole sleeve of the trunk, all this soft tissue that I can touch at the front and the back and the sides here, is involved in the function of the arm, the function here of reaching – which I am doing for you, which doing on my part allows you to more clearly feel it – but also in gesturing or manipulations of every kind. You want all of this to be involved when the arm is used, which involvement supports the arm and gives it direction.

'In addition, all this soft tissue engages the trunk, the ribcage particularly. The ribcage is rather like a concertina. In a similar way to its action in your breathing where the ribcage expands and contracts, when you reach or gesture or manipulate, the ribcage rightly expands and contracts as it is involved in the arm's movements.

'So think of all of that. Thinking informs self-sensing and moving and the nervous system will make the connections as you give it more and more stimulus.

'Greater freedom of the ribcage allows for greater suppleness of the spine at its core, which suppleness allows for an improved freedom of the head at the top of the spine.

'Now sitting here, your legs are clearly directed forward from the pelvis, the pelvis being the bottom of the back. Similarly, the legs are going apart because the legs are shaped rather like canes whose handle points outwards from the pelvis at the hip joint. You want to agree with the natural design and release the legs away from each other and the knees forward. You don't pull them apart; you wish them apart. And if they don't seem to or you can't feel it, keep with thinking it anyway.

'Now come to the lower leg, ankle and foot. The lower leg is two bones that can rotate around each other like the bones of the forearm and they stand on the ankle, whose seven bones work together rather like a ball-bearing. The ankle rests on the foot, which is structured like a tripod, where the feet of the tripod are the ball of the big toe, the ball of the little toe and the heel. So the foot relative to the lower leg can potentially move freely at the ankle a little like the hand at the wrist.

'Because we bind our feet in shoes and walk primarily on flat surfaces that offer little challenge of adaptation to the foot and ankle, the mobility of the ankle tends to be compromised in almost everyone.

'Now let's come back to the head–neck relationship, the first link in the chain of the primary control. Your thinking should always be returning there, and then to all the rest, all at once, one after another.

'So, you free the head–neck relationship by freeing the neck; you free the back, the arms from the back, the legs from the trunk, releasing the feet into the floor and follow the head into standing.

'Come and lie on your back on the table with your head on these books and your legs bent, your feet standing, in what we call the semi-supine position. This shape Alexander called a position of mechanical advantage because it puts the major muscle groups in their mid-range where they are most easily left alone and from which one is most ready to act.

'Although you are lying down, we are still working with the organization of movement in the actural dynamic. Only here we are removing the requirement of most of that musculature to work so that we can facilitate its improved organization while in a more passive state, which improved organization we can then bring back to in-gravity activity.

'So again you come back with your mind altogether to the head and its freedom on the top of the spine. You allow it to come out so that the spine can lengthen.

'Let me take the arm.

'I'm supporting the arm here by holding your hand and here by supporting your scapula. So you are letting it go from the ribcage, as you let the head go from the neck. Perhaps you notice that it is easier to let the arm alone here in lying down than when you were standing.

'Let the ribcage come along, letting it go from the spine. There. Now the spine is freer to lengthen following the head.

'The same with this arm. You let the arm release from the back, from the ribcage, which is the back, and this release of the arm serves to release the back. All of this widens the back and allows the back as a whole to lengthen.

'The work with the legs is similar.

'As a part of the skeletal structure the leg comes out of the bottom of the back at the hip joint. You wish it free at the hip joint. It is also true that, a little like the shoulder girdle, the pelvic girdle plays a part in the use of the leg. You want to wish for that engagement of the pelvis with the leg and include that in your understanding of what a leg is. You want to release the pelvic girdle from the back.

'The leg as a function comes out of the centre and away from the head via the back. Let me explain.

'The main flexor of the leg, the psoas muscle, originates up here, at the front of the lumbar spine. So, functionally speaking, the leg starts up here in the centre of the body. The main extensors of the leg are the hamstrings and gluteals which work in conjunction with the paraspinals that run up to the back of the head. So, functionally speaking, the leg comes out of the centre and away from the head via the back. And I look to feel that and you want to feel for that and to think that as I take the leg here.

'And the same with the other leg. I am taking the weight of the leg so you can leave it alone.

'Now when we come back to the head you notice that it is freer with respect to the neck and that the back lengthens even more. This is because the body works integrally and when you free one part the whole thing is freer.

'And so we can now come back to the arms…then back to the head…back to the legs…and so on…until we get the most we are going to get on the table in terms of renewed freedom for action. In a moment then we can come back to standing.

'Let me get you off the table. All you have to do is continue to think your directions while I levitate you.

'Come back to the stool, standing as though to sit.

'So you will notice that you feel lighter, taller and broader. The lightness is a perception founded on the softening of the tendons caused by the release of the muscles throughout the system. You also are taller and broader.

'Remarkably, though the muscles are more released throughout the system, you are not slumped and collapsed but rather more up and functionally stronger. This is the magic of the Technique.

'Now we want to associate this renewed global buoyancy with functioning in the actural dynamic.

'Again, give your directions relative to freeing the neck, releasing the head forward and up from the top of the spine, allowing the back to lengthen and widen, the shoulders to release apart and the legs to release forward and away. And then consider again how to fold into sitting while keeping all those directions going.

'Simply allow the knees and hips to bend and stop here, part way to the stool. Allow the shoulder girdle to float and the arms to hang from the ribcage via the shoulder girdle. Let the head continue to float from the top of the neck, the whole back including the head to come up and back from the legs, the heels down, the knees forward and away, the arms releasing out from the top of the back, via the shoulder girdle, up and back with the back in the direction that the clavicles point.

'Let me take your arm here. Allow it to come up freely into a gesture like beholding. Then let's come to the other arm and do the same. Allow the arms to come up and back as extensions of the back, and allow them to release outwards even to the fingertips, widening the back.

'Think up and back here, up and back as though you were releasing up against my hand pressing on your back here.

'And now, letting the arms down, unfold at the knees and the hips, releasing the legs out of the bottom of the back and thereby the heels into the floor, and come again to your full natural height.

'Again, folding the legs at the knees and hips and releasing the body in all directions upwards and outwards, come back into sitting.

'One more time, think your directions, releasing yourself up from the place of support and out from the centre, the head leading the whole release into freedom, and follow the head into standing, and go for a little walk.'

A SECOND
(IMPOSSIBLE) LESSON

'So what we are working with here is the organization of movement in the actural dynamic. I am working on the outside and you on the inside.

'As I have said, the primary control is not a thing in space or process through time but the manner of action. You can recognize it in whatever it is you recognize when you differentiate the organization of human movement from that of, say, an ape. That is the primary control as perceived from the outside. We are seeking to facilitate your finding it on the inside.

'The primary control is the organization of all of yourself, which can be apprehended all at once, as a gestalt, and controlled all at once because the nervous system indeed organizes mass movements.

'Alexander discovered that the organization of movement is sequential, instant and integrated: that the head's freedom on the neck is first in the sequence of free movement, followed by freedom of the back, the centre and the five cardinal lines.

'With my words and hands I encourage you to free the neck to let the head go forward and up from the top of the spine to let the back lengthen and widen to let the shoulders release up and away and the legs to release forward and away; with my hands I help a little here and here and here to encourage that freeing sequence; and you are to conform yourself to all that to the best of your growing ability.

'It is always the same thing you are doing whenever you decide to do it: the exercise of consciousness in the context of the coordination of movement.

'The details of the practice in each person's case emerge more and more in time. At first, you become aware of what we might describe as the gross parts: the head, the neck, the trunk, the legs and the arms. In the beginning, people are barely aware of the pelvis. As the grosser patterns of contraction and those in the peripheral parts are broken down a little, subtler patterns emerge, and patterns closer to the axial line and the centre.

'Notice how much is going on inside of you.

'You want to leave the legs alone here, letting them be forward and away in their direction from the pelvis. And let the arms here float up off the top of the ribcage via the shoulder girdle. Let the head here float on top and the back follow. And now, keeping those directions going, follow the head into standing.

'All the words I use – "free, release, relax, let be, allow, let go, let float, drop, open, send such and such away", even "follow" or "involve" – are the same instruction.

'We have to use conscious means because otherwise unconscious habits continue. This would be obvious were you learning to play a musical instrument. You can't learn to play a musical instrument unconsciously. Similarly with the instrument that is your body. Of course, with respect to the body, you have spent however many years practicing with it poorly and developing habits of practice that first must be undone.

'So let the neck go a little more here so that the head can be a little lighter on top. And think of allowing the whole spine from the head to the pelvis to release freely up out of the legs, and allowing the whole back to widen. Alexander once described the lengthening and widening of the back as smoothing out a crumpled piece of paper. Let the widening and lengthening of the back extend into the releasing of the arms and legs out from the centre of you and away from each other. Let the whole frontal line from the hips through the belly, stomach, chest and throat open and release upwards.

'And, keeping all that thinking alive, allow yourself to fold at the hips, knees and ankles and lightly return to sitting.

'Now with my hands on your sides here feel the width of the ribcage. And here at the base of the ribs feel the depth of the ribcage.

And here, the belly, the bottom of the ribcage. And here under the shoulders, feel the top of the ribcage. And let it all expand freely, that is, without your doing anything to make it happen. Let the arms and legs release outwards. Let the head be free on top. And let yourself tilt forward and back on the sitting bones. And again, follow the head into standing.

'Come to the table.

'Sitting on the edge of the table, again think your directions. And keeping that thinking going, bring the feet to stand on the table. Let the arms go, let the spine lengthen, and release yourself backwards vertebra by vertebra onto the table and your head onto the books.

'Let the head's freedom from the neck allow the back to lengthen here. Let the shoulders come up from the top of the back to give more space for the back.

'Let the right arm's freedom from the ribcage allow the back to widen here. Let the space created for the ribcage serve to spread the ribcage like a concertina.

'The same with the left arm. Let it too release off the ribcage and give more space for the ribcage to do what it will do when it has more freedom, which is to expand.

'Come to the left leg. Let its freedom via the pelvic girdle allow the low back to lengthen and widen here. Let the ankle release, the knee, the hip, the leg drawing on the pelvis to draw on the back.

'The same with the right leg. Let the whole leg undo and come out more and more as I take its weight here and straighten it, and also as I bend it back into standing.

'Back to the head on top to coordinate the whole process of expansion in all directions.

'And we will keep at that a little longer until we've got all the expansion we are likely to get out of you for today...

'So let me get you off the table. Again all you have to do is continue to think your directions while I levitate you.

'Come back to the stool, standing prepared to sit.

'Let the head release up and the back lengthen, allow the ankles, knees and hips to fold, the knees going out, the hips and back going back, and, going up to go down, pause here in monkey.

'Let this arm float up and extend from and widen the back here, and this one, here. Feel the dynamism of this pose and its ease and strength.

'And feel my pushing down on your shoulders here. Feel the buoyancy of the whole system, spring-loaded. I could be standing on your shoulders and it would be easy.

'Now, going up to go down, come into sitting.

'We'll place this chair here with its back to you.

'Let me take your hand and arm, letting the back widen as the arm floats up and out. With the fingers straight-ish rest them on the front of the back of the chair here. Bring the thumb into contact on the back, your fingers and thumb working like a bird's beak. Let the wrist be directed inwards from the elbow and the elbow outwards both from the wrist and from the spine. Let the whole arm float up off the back. Let some of its weight pass into the chair.

'The same with this arm. Let this arm widen the back as the arm floats up and out. And again with the fingers straight-ish rest them on the front of the back of the chair here. And bring the thumb into contact with the back. Let the wrist be directed inwards and the elbow outwards. Let the whole arm float up off the back. Let some of its weight pass into the chair.

'Let the elbows here lightly release up and out.

'Now let me tilt you forward and back on your sitting bones as you let the arms float.

'Continue to think your directions – neck free, head forward and up, back lengthening and widening, knees forward and away, shoulders up and away.

'Now let me take your arms down. And come back into standing.

'Keeping these directions going, just think about coming onto your toes. Even though the heels will be moving upwards, continue to release them out of the back. And continue to direct the pelvis back, even as it will move forward in space.

'Come then onto your toes and notice how clear is the buoyancy of the whole structure.

'Then return to your heels and notice the more subtle buoyancy now of the structure – through the whole spine and trunk, the legs and the arches of the feet.

'Again come onto your toes while you keep all the thinking alive, and here gently come up a little higher and then lower and higher and lower, and notice the ease and lightness possible in the action when the thinking is clear.

'Now let just one heel down. And then come up with it again. Then the other. And then come up with it again. And the first one down again. And then as you take the other down, bring the first up, and gently and lightly, begin to walk in place.

'OK, and come lightly back onto your heels and lightly into the chair.

'Allow yourself to rock lightly and slightly forward and back on the sitting bones while keeping the back released and buoyant.

'Then come back into standing and go for a walk.'

TEACHING REMARKS

- We don't need to fight gravity: we won several million years ago.

- If you move the shoulders back from where I've taken them, it is because you have a preferred position that feels right. That can't work to effect useful change. It doesn't matter what I do with you. It's how you respond. However the body is positioned is unimportant. We are not working with positioning or structure but with the manner of action. Imagine if you were bending down under a kitchen sink with a wrench to get at a bolt behind the drainpipe. It's not likely to feel right or be a position of preference but you still have to think out a response to the challenge while allowing the body to remain free.

- You don't want to hold what you feel to be the 'right' position, which holding by definition stiffens you and prevents the freedom we are after.

- Always do less. Minimizing effort in the midst of any action or position is an essential element of inhibition.

- Whenever you notice you are doing something to try to get it right, stop doing that thing, and see what emerges.

- If we were not holding on to it we would not have to learn to let it go.

- You don't want to berate yourself if you notice that you're reacting because you may then associate negative feeling with moments of self-discovery. Each of us is constantly going wrong. Walter

Carrington once remarked that, once you begin the Technique, you are continually discovering thereafter where you are going wrong. The more you notice yourself going wrong, the more you let it go, the more you direct, the sooner will pass these symptoms that you are suffering. The symptoms are a function in part of the infrequency of your self-awareness. There will always be new things to notice, more subtle things, because, as you become more and more *sensitive* to the subtleties of your faulty reaction, you become more and more sensitive to the *subtleties* of your faulty reaction.

• You cannot already know what you are going to learn.

• (In response to a comment by a student that he felt good for two days following a lesson.) The feeling is a consequence of your improving coordination. That manner of organizing your movement in such a way that you were feeling especially good is not something you can ordinarily access. What we are seeking to grow as a somatic capability, to bring to 'conscious control', is the intelligence that is informing that improved self-organization. It is that coordination that is subject to your use. The feeling is not subject to your use and that is why end-gaining can't work.

ENDS AND MEANS

In Goddard Binkley's diary of lessons with Alexander he reports that, during one lesson, he questioned Alexander's criticism of the work of Charles Neale, a graduate of the first training, saying that Neale was getting excellent results with his students. Alexander's remark in response was something like, 'That's what I said: he's not teaching the Alexander Technique': because the Technique is not defined by the goals achieved by one's actions but by one's manner of action (Binkley 1993).

• (In response to a pupil who objected to my occasional use of 'good' and 'right', connoting, he felt, moral judgment.) If this work were to be part of a spiritual practice, say, in the manner of yoga, then, as somatic learning it would follow and follow from moral responsibilities just as *asana* and *pranayama* come after the *yamas* and *niyamas*. As a practicing Jew, following the Ten Commandments would come first; as a Christian, obeying Jesus' Two Laws: 'Love God with all your soul, all your heart, all your mind and all your strength, and your neighbour as yourself'; as a Buddhist, adhering to the Five Precepts. Here the words 'good' and 'right' apply rather to the quality of your attention, thinking, inhibition, direction, self-sensing and movement.

- You can know that you are getting it wrong because ultimately only you are responsible for this functional limitation. By then projecting the directions with respect to the best organization of the primary control, you give the nervous system a right imagined experience to remake your wrong actual experience. This works because the nervous system has been shown to respond similarly to imagined and actual experiences.

- The power of movement comes from the potential energy provided by our radical uprightness, not from the pelvis.

- Stretching muscles can't re-educate them. Stretching can't even be done voluntarily and directly. Muscles only contract. Thus, you can only consciously contract or not contract a muscle. Conscious use of muscles is required for their re-education.

- Alexander discouraged pupils from closing their eyes or staring during lessons as he believed these activities to be trance states that slowed the progress of learning to use the Technique in waking life. The essence of trance is the binding of consciousness to conditions. In contrast, both the means and goal of the Technique is free attention.

Manipulations

EVOLUTIONS

Alexander observed a primary global bodily pattern of self-contraction. Hanna and Feldenkrais identified the secondary patterns of anxiety, effort and protection, each of which manifests globally. Obvious too are a pattern of collapse and the necessary compensating patterns involved in 'holding oneself up'. Alexander also noticed other local patterns. One that he mentions in his own case was a habit that he learned as an actor of 'taking hold of the floor with the feet'. (Although Alexander does not explicitly say so one can guess that taking hold of the floor with the feet is a bad idea.)

The primary control, as the root 'shaping' of human movement, is not readily accessible to our attention or control. Because of this the Technique typically works in simple positions and movements. More complex movements are in general too difficult to organize by and for a student while maintaining the right use of the primary control. Positions of mechanical advantage, by their very organization, serve this end simply. Beyond these there is an increasingly challenging range of manipulations that, with persistent application, can bring about a resolution of dysfunctional patterns and the emergence of natural grace.

POSITIONS OF MECHANICAL ADVANTAGE

The three positions of mechanical advantage are semi-supine, sitting with the hands on the lap and 'monkey' and its variations. A particularly dynamic way to work in semi-supine is to lie with a foam roller or tightly rolled blanket along the length of the spine from the base of the neck to the tailbone, the head supported accordingly. This brings to the position an added challenge of balancing as in standing and discourages mind-wandering and mere relaxing in the position; it highlights the spine and encourages the settling, release and lengthening of the spine and the consequent widening of the back; and it can help to open the frontal line. After several minutes using the roller thus, one should tip carefully from it and continue semi-supine on the floor.

In sitting there is an added challenge for a person with strong ideas about good posture or sitting straight. Good use is not about being straight or holding a position. Freedom, adaptability and buoyancy are the goals of practice, which emerge through self-exploration and evocation.

Freedom is achieved only through conscious means because we are bound unconsciously to dysfunctional patterns. Were we already free, the directions would manifest spontaneously. Until then we consciously evoke those directions, served at first by our teacher, in order to resolve the patterning that interferes with the inherent directions.

In sitting we want a dynamic coordination. It is useful in the practice of sitting – and in monkey and variations – to have an arrangement of full-length mirrors in which to observe oneself from a variety of angles without disturbance to the orientation of the head, especially from the sides and from the back. Using mirrors, one must be careful not to correct oneself directly according to a preconceived notion of what is a right appearance, but rather use the observations as redundant information by which to corroborate and calibrate one's self-sensing.

In monkey one can stimulate greater sensory information and motor challenge by deepening the bending of the knees or changing the angle of the trunk. The greater the tone, the greater the sensory information stimulated and the greater the challenges and effects on one's control, self-sensing and self-organization.

Standing is the radically upright form of monkey. It is possible to be virtually relaxed in standing, the pose supported reflexively. In standing, some people tend to pull the knees back, over-straightening them, or push the hips forward, thereby swaying the back forward, which contradicts Nature's design.

These developing positions give increasing sensory information about the best organization of the primary control while facilitating that best organization. The verbal directions provide a clear handle to which to attach one's intention. They are to be used to facilitate intention and may in time be given up so that one can connect one's thinking directly to the sensorimotor event. Some teachers use images such as balloons and strings attached to the head and so on. If one begins with such images they should be soon discarded as dissociation from, rather than integration with, physical reality is probable.

While it is true that the primary control as a motor concept is a feed-forward sensorimotor image that one is projecting or towards which one is 'feeling' it is an image that is linked to physical correlates.

ELEMENTAL MOVEMENTS

When working in a position of mechanical advantage one can gently experiment with elemental movements: forward or lateral flexion, extension or rotation of the trunk; flexion, extension, abduction, adduction or rotation of the limbs; thrusting, pushing, pulling, lifting, gesturing or reaching; shifting, twisting or turning at any of the joints of the body including the spine; even stepping. Combinations of any of these may also be tried. Such movements will enhance both the quality and quantity of self-sensing and will challenge coordination.

A potential liability in practice is the tendency for movement to be minimized and the transfer of improved sensorimotor competence to activities in daily life to be made poorly. Alexander (2001) defined the primary control as 'a certain relativity of the head with the neck and of the head–neck relationship with the back and with the rest of the body', a definition that does not clearly account for coordinated movement and the play and direction of forces. By working with a variety of elemental movements the potential problem of state-specific learning is diminished.

There is only limited conscious control possible in the context of the complexities of daily life. By practicing with the building blocks of elemental movements one provides oneself a growing foundation for all movements.

APPLICATIONS

One can go on to what are called applications, which bring the Technique into simple activities. To work with applications one must continue to minimize one's reliance on 'doing and feeling' because feeling can only be relied upon when it is reliable. Thus, in order to work with applications, one must already have a grasp of the primary control and more reliable sensory appreciation. Many applications have been explored in detail in Judith Leibowitz's book, *The Alexander Technique*. Applications involve the simplest actions such as reaching, gesturing, bending, turning the head or the trunk, stepping, carrying light items, sitting or standing with the hands on a table top, speaking, holding a pen, leaning, pulling on a handle, turning a dial, pushing an object and other basic activities in the context of which one can practice the fundamentals of the Technique.

ILLUSTRATIONS: WRITING AND LIFTING

Writing involves sitting, looking down and using the arm and hand as manipulative functions. Like many everyday activities it is a complex action that seems simple. Sitting is an organization of the whole system in the actural dynamic. Looking down involves mainly a tonic coordination of the spine. Using the arm and hand to manipulate an object is a coordinated movement of the arm supported and stabilized by the trunk.

Sit at a desk and place the feet under the knees, the arms resting on the desk. Allow the head to release from the neck, the back to lengthen and widen, the legs to release forward and away, and the arms to release from the back. Release yourself upwards, following the head, from the place of support on the chair under the sitting bones and outwards from the centre via the five cardinal lines. Don't slump but don't sit up straight.

Hinge forward on the sitting bones, allowing the trunk to be supple, neither rigid nor floppy. Keep the legs released at the hips even as you incline forward. Drop the eyes to the writing paper. Release the back of the neck only enough for effective viewing of the writing material. In the same way as the sitting bones are shaped like the rockers of a rocking chair, the bottom of the skull where it rests on the atlas vertebra is similarly shaped and rocks forward to tilt the head down.

Take the pen, folding the extended fingers and thumb on the instrument lightly, bearing its weight as though with the arm and back. Imagine holding a hollow eggshell or soap bubble near the midpoint of the digits. Understand that it is the hand and arm that does the writing. Then do the writing, unconcerned about its appearance.

Lifting an object, a large box for example, involves standing and bending and the use of the body with the arms as a weight-bearing function and the hands as grasping functions.

Stand with the feet a little more than shoulder width apart as close as is practicable to the object. Give your directions. Don't slump but don't stand straight.

Keep the legs released at the hips as you fold into 'monkey'. Let the arms hang freely as you deepen the bend letting the knees go comfortably apart until reaching for the object is easy. Take the object firmly, with the palms of the hands making clear contact. Keeping the object as close to your centre of gravity as possible and, releasing the neck and leading with the head, the weight of yourself and the object directed through the apices of the feet, unfold into standing.

Any activity or action sequence can be so treated as an application, broken down into its elements and synthesized into a whole, a laboratory for self-study and experimentation with the directions of right use.

BREATHING

Senior and central to the organization of movement is the function of the breath. Alexander's first description of the Technique was as a method of respiratory re-education. At the start of his work, he was known as 'the breathing man' because the Technique serves to free and integrate the entire trunk wherein breathing takes place.

Breathing is generated reflexively by a coordinated use of some sixty muscles. In the inspiration phase of this complex action the ribcage hinges as a whole forward and out at the joint of the sternum and manubrium in a manner similar to the initial lifting of a bucket handle from the side of the bucket; the ribcage widens and lengthens via a separation of the ribs like the opening of Venetian blinds; the diaphragm, an umbrella-like tendonous sheet that separates the thoracic and the abdominal cavities, is drawn downward like a piston, pushing the abdomen and pelvic floor down and out and widening the floating ribs; the upper ribcage is stabilized or lifted via musculature attaching the top ribs to the front of the neck; and the twelfth rib is stabilized or drawn down lengthening the bottom of the ribcage like a concertina. All of this produces an enlargement of and partial vacuum in the thoracic cavity into which is drawn ambient air. In the expiration phase of this process all these actions are relaxed.

Respiration happens spontaneously and properly when one 'gets out of the way' and allows oneself 'to be breathed'.

Neither the nasal passages, oral cavity, throat, trachea nor any part of the lungs are actively involved in inspiration or expiration. The physical work is accomplished by the diaphragm musculature, the sternalis and intercostal muscles, some smaller trunk muscles located in the back, the scalenes and the quadratus lumborum. The net effect of these reflex muscular efforts is an increase in the interior volume of the ribcage to the inside of which the lungs are glued. The lungs thus expand with the increase in volume of the thoracic cavity. Because of their sponge-like constitution the lungs absorb air passively into their microscopic pockets, the alveoli. Attention may be given inwardly to the expansion of the thoracic cavity whose envelope is the diaphragm and the ribcage.

Alexander observed that each of us tends to narrow, shorten and compress the trunk, preventing the easy expansion of the thoracic cavity in breathing. In addition, many of us also contract the abdominal wall from anxiety or in conformity to fashion or as armouring. This contraction of the belly wall inhibits the ability to take a full in-breath by compressing the contents of the abdomen, thereby preventing the easy downward movement of the diaphragm – the greater part of the breathing function. This may oblige inspiration to be accomplished through the lifting of the upper chest as in exertion, a manner of breathing that can contribute to the gasping for air during speaking, to anxiety and to asthma.

THE WHISPERED 'AH'

Ideally speaking involves the controlled use of expiration while vocalizing. Speech interrupts the natural flow of the breath. Alexander developed the whispered 'ah' as an indirect foundation evolution to serve the improvement of breathing and speaking. Like other evolutions, we address the basics of a function to facilitate an improvement in the complex use of the function.

The whispered 'ah' serves to relax the musculature of the face, throat, diaphragm, belly and vocal apparatus in the context of breathing and speaking. The 'ah' sound is in some sense the matrix of all sounds as monkey is the matrix of all action in gravity. The 'ah' sound provides advantageous conditions for observing and releasing oneself in the context of vocalizing as monkey and positions of mechanical advantage provide advantageous conditions for observing and releasing oneself in the context of movement in gravity. All speech shapes the 'ah' sound as all movement shapes monkey.

To produce the best sound, one relaxes the neck, throat and oral cavity, releasing the jaw, relaxing the face and tongue and allowing a controlled release of the trunk in expiration.

In normal waking life, the tongue rests on the bottom of the mouth, its tip touching the upper palate at the root of the upper front teeth, the mouth lightly closed. Tension in the tongue can be allied with tension in the neck.

To begin the procedure you allow the natural cycling of the breath. You are not to take a deep inspiration or interrupt the breathing but rather begin with the natural expiration. You allow the air to escape via a whisper through the opened mouth and relaxed throat and neck, easing the breath out with a controlled compression of the abdominal region, expelling the air slowly via a slight drawing up of the pelvic floor and an ascending compression of the frontal musculature from the pubic bone to the intercostal arch.

When the expiration reaches a natural end, without any squeezing of the trunk, relax the jaw so that it spontaneously closes. Then relax the frontal line and allow the return of the breath, continuing the practice with the next expiration.

This procedure takes patient relaxed observation and can be repeated at will. As one gains competence in this, one can try the 'ah' sound with vocalization or the addition of soft consonantal stops at the end or start.

THE TARZAN BREATH

For some of us the breathing is initially too compromised to allow the release of the breath cycle directly or to work effectively with the whispered 'ah'. In *The Miracle of the Breath*, Andy Caponigro suggests a couple of manipulations of the breathing pattern that can serve to break up the kinds of obstructive patterns that afflict some of us.

The first, which he calls the Tarzan breath, involves exhaling with a loud 'ah' vocalization while pounding the chest like a charging ape sufficiently strongly to cause a breaking of the voice, doing this through many breath cycles, then following this with a period of simple observation of the breathing, allowing the manipulation to have its effect, which can be an evening, calming, opening or fulfilling of the respiratory cycle.

The second manipulation he describes involves a panting style of breathing but with the mouth closed, again repeated through many breath cycles. This too can serve to break up obstructions in the respiratory pattern and allow the natural pattern to better establish itself. Again, following this manipulation, one is to merely observe the breathing and notice what effects emerge from the process.

Both these manipulations can begin to make more obvious the interferences with the natural pattern, which may then be addressed more ably with inhibition.

HANDS ON THE BACK OF A CHAIR

'Hands on the back of a chair' is an evolution that exemplifies the Alexander approach to sensorimotor learning in its address to a foundation process as a means to serve more complex processes. What is important in this evolution is the use of the arms and hands as an extension of the back and as a function of the whole body. At the same time that it is to be accomplished as a global process the local details must be put together piece by piece.

'Hands on the back of a chair' can be done in sitting or in monkey. The hands are to perch with the four fingers and the thumb closing on the chair back, extended from the first joint of the digits rather like a bird's beak. The wrists are to point towards each other, and the elbows away from both the wrists and the trunk via the shoulder girdle. The front is to open and the back to widen drawing the elbows apart, creating elasticity in the trunk and limbs.

One may have a sense and idea of some of the weight of the arms dropping into the chair via the fingers so that some of the arms' weight is thereby released from the trunk, allowing the trunk to further widen and release upwards following the head.

Hinging the trunk forward and backward on the sitting bones in sitting or from the hips in monkey will further free the arms from the ribcage and at the wrists via a relative conjugate movement of the proximal part, the trunk, relative to the distal parts, the arms.

Elaborations of this evolution can involve elemental movements such as pushing or pulling the chair-back to rock the chair on its legs, slowly flapping the elbows, lifting the chair, or 'stretching' the back of the chair via a widening of the back.

Strictly speaking, monkey with the hands on the back of a chair is the only position of mechanical advantage, the trunk and legs most advantageously organized for action and the arms and hands for manipulations. The net effect of this evolution when mastered is the virtual taking over of the anti-gravity response and manipulative functions by the extensor and abductor musculature allowing the release of the frontal musculature for the most effortless cycling of the breath.

ALTERNATIVE APPROACHES TO THE ORGANIZATION OF FUNCTION

One approach to the organization of an action pattern advocated by early practitioners of the Technique, and probably drawn from Alexander's own practice in his years of exploration, is in a step-by-step linear style.

It would proceed in the following way.

In standing, say, you first give yourself the direction, 'Let the neck be free,' and then check in your sensory experience for some effect.

Follow that by giving yourself the directions, 'Let the neck be free, to let the head revolve forward and up from the top of the spine,' and again check in your sensory experience for an effect.

Then follow that by giving yourself the directions, 'Let the neck be free, to let the head revolve forward and up from the top of the spine, to let the back lengthen,' and again check in your sensory experience for an effect.

Then follow that by giving yourself the directions, 'Let the neck be free, to let the head revolve forward and up from the top of the spine, to let the back lengthen and widen,' and check in your sensory experience for an effect.

You would follow each set of directions with a repetition of that entire preceding set of directions and then adding the next step until you have completed the entire set of preparatory directions: 'Let the neck be free, to let the head revolve forward and up from the top of the spine, to let the back lengthen and widen, to let one shoulder release away from the centre, to let that release extend through the arm to the wrist and on to the tips of the fingers, to let the other shoulder release away from the centre, to let that release extend through the arm to the wrist and on to the tips of the fingers, to let the hips release apart, to let the legs release forward and away,' and after each step in the set of directions, 'looking' into your sensory experience for an effect before proceeding to the next step in the directions.

At this point in the procedure you are prepared to do a physical action.

If that action were to perform the evolution, hands-on-the-back-of-a-chair in 'monkey', you would then give yourself the set of directions, 'Let the neck be free, to let the head revolve forward and up from the top of the spine, to let the back lengthen and widen, to let one shoulder release away from the centre, to let that release extend through the arm to the wrist and on to the tips of the fingers, to let the other shoulder release away from the centre, to let that release extend through the arm to the wrist and on to the tips of the fingers, to let the legs release forward and away, to let the knees bend.'

Then you would repeat the entire set of directions to this stage, adding then the direction to let one arm extend out to take hold of the back of the chair, followed by the direction to let the other arm extend out to take hold of the back of the chair.

This description of such an approach to the practice illustrates the nature of the concentrated mental work that may be required to transform the quality of a function working on one's own. And it is a good practice as it effectively disciplines both self-awareness and the will as they are used in the Technique. While a skilled teacher can often, with his hands and in a few minutes, effect this whole series of integrated patterns, practice in this fashion with any simple action pattern is useful for one's learning and serves to reinforce the effect of lessons.

What is assumed and then practiced in the Alexander Technique is the prior freedom of attention, which is to be enacted in, via and as the body. The application of that attention through any action pattern can be practiced in greater and greater detail in order to refine attention and learn to notice smaller and smaller differences.

We have access to our motor function via the muscles and to our structure and the organization of function via perception and motor concepts. All of these comprise our soma or somatic experience, the purview of the Technique.

Much of the musculature of the shoulders, back, ribcage, face and neck invests into the aponeurosis of the skull or skullcap. The skull rests on the atlas vertebra.

This is probably the origin of the myth of Atlas who supports the World. Douglas Harding, who wrote the book, *On Having No Head* (2006), describes his realization in 'having no head' as one of 'becoming the world' that 'appears' in and as one's experience 'above the shoulders'. Tom Hanna was saying something like that in his one-time remark, 'The soma is me,' the 'perceptual body'.

So begin by resting your attention on, or begin to think of, the head and its support in the area of atlanto-occipital junction, whatever that is in your current experience and best intelligence.

You're going to go through the whole body, in detail, from head to core to extremities, and release it and organize it in that release. You must take some time to do it properly and you can take as much time as you want.

Bring your attention then to the neck – and the face, throat, shoulders and the top of the back – and direct it all to release in a way that allows the head to, as it were, 'float' from and revolve forward in its floating from the top of the spine, allowing the whole spine to lengthen and so the back altogether including the depth of the ribcage to widen – and do all of this to the best of your current ability now, while you're reading. (The experience, both of that organization and the 'feeling' of that organization, may be found in somatic 'memory' from work in your lessons with a teacher.)

And you can go back sometimes and, in going back, you may notice differences in your experience next time.

The head 'floats' up and revolves forward from the top of the spine, lengthening the whole spine and trunk and widening the trunk. Because most of the ribs are fixed at the sternum and spine they expand mostly at the sides of you. The last two pairs of so-called 'floating' ribs on either side just above the waist can widen even more.

As the spine lengthens with the breathing, right up to the head, the myofascia that connect the head to the shoulders, let the shoulders float away from the back and ribcage. See if you can find that or allow for that.

Relax the muscles of the face and the eyes; the neck, the sides and back and the frontal and core musculature of the neck – some of the hyoid group of muscles in the neck that serve the function of the tongue are almost horizontal to the spinal axis: and so relax the tongue; release the shoulders too and even then the arms and hands all the way to the fingertips; the musculature of the ribcage connecting through to the pelvis; and the whole back in its length down to the pelvis and its width, which is the width of the ribcage, and so its depth – its depth is what widens.

The breathing, which is central to the body, relaxes the body in all its directions and dimensions: via the head and tail and then via the arms and legs and via the widening of the trunk, the whole thing expanding – from the core of you – relaxing into expansion and relaxing into non-expansion.

Some teachers of the Technique apply themselves almost exclusively to the fundamentals of the primary control: the head-neck-spine. And that, in itself, is a beginning. Many include the back: the head-neck-back; some, the head-neck-trunk; a few, the head-neck-spine-trunk-core – which is where we've gotten to so far.

Let's go on.

You can be standing or sitting while you do this. It may be okay to be lying down if you were, say, lying semi-supine under a glass table with the book open to this page, even on a roller to bring the spine into focus.

Go gently back now and slowly check the freedom of the head-neck-spine-trunk-core, in detail, step by step from the head, skullcap and face, the neck all over and inside, the spine, the width and depth of the back and the width of the ribcage, and the breathing, the ribs expanding especially at the sides and right down to the bottom.

And then let's go to the shoulders or shoulder girdle, the clavicles releasing outwards and, as it were, drawing along the whole chest; do this slowly – you direct that – and the scapulae the same, releasing outwards and drawing along the width of the trunk – and you direct that – and then the upper arms and elbows and forearms, inside and outside and altogether, the wrists, the hands, the palms and the backs of the hands, and the digits right out to their tips, the whole of both hands: the whole of both arms then through their linkage from the pelvis through the ribcage to the ends of the thumbs and fingers.

You can go through one arm at a time. Try it that way too and both arms together. And then the legs the same way: the pelvic girdle releasing out of the back and axial trunk at the sacroiliac joints, revolving back over the hips; the thighs to the knees, all of these releasing, the lower legs to the ankles at the apices of the feet, the tripods of the feet to the heels and to all the toes and the length of the toes: the legs and arms released and directed then altogether outwards from the core, front and back and sides and through and through.

And then you can go back to the top and repeat all of this if you like.

OK, now try sitting with a couple of small objects before you at a distance beyond easy reach – lemons, oranges, glasses or eggs will do – and again go through the above sequence in a calm address to the release and organization of all of yourself.

Then consider the right arm and its connection through your centre to and from the right foot and so, to reach for one of the objects before you, the right hand leads, the fingers extended, the whole apparatus following link by link in a flowing expansive movement and the trunk beginning to move towards the object, the centre of the body drawn into the movement and that moving through space, grounded on the chair, the movement 'powered' by the potential energy of uprightness and supported by the coordinated work of the whole-bodily musculature, all the while quietly breathing – and coming to take hold of one of the objects with the whole hand, the palm making clear contact and the fingers and thumbs extending around it gently.

Then consider the left arm connected through the centre from the right foot.

To reach for the other object before you, again the hand leads, the fingers extended, the whole apparatus following link by link in a flowing expansive movement and the trunk beginning to move towards the object, the centre of the body drawn into the movement and moving in a path through the space, grounded on the chair, the movement 'powered' by the potential energy of uprightness and supported by the coordinated effort of the whole-bodily musculature, all the while quietly breathing – and coming to take hold of the second object with the whole hand, the palm making clear contact and the fingers and thumbs extending around it gently.

Now, using this approach, let's try something in standing.

Again go back and slowly check the freedom of the head-neck-spine-trunk-core, in detail, step by step from the head, skullcap and face, the neck all over and inside, the spine, the width and depth of the back and the width of the ribcage, and the breathing, the ribs expanding especially at the sides and right down to the bottom. Go through the sequence, calmly addressing the release and organization of all of yourself.

Let the arms release via the shoulders up and away from the ribcage, the chest and the back, the legs releasing into the floor and out of the floor.

Now, lean forward slightly via the ankles from the floor.

To take a step, which foot would move and which would 'stand'? When your tilting forward lightens the body in space, pause.

Now the head always already leads this and every movement; the moving knee will lead the stepping action; the centre of gravity in the vital centre will glide forward in space; the arms will begin to swing forward from their links at the shoulder joints; the legs will articulate at the hip joints and knees. The body will flow forward with virtually no effort, moved by the potential energy of the high centre of gravity from the floor under the 'standing' foot. Allow yourself to be breathed and release yourself into walking.

You may find that the feet track more or less in a line and therefore remain more or less under the centre of gravity which moves in a smooth forward line through space.

Consider playing with each of the above approaches and also the general approach described in the section 'Applications' above at various times during the day in the carrying out of any simple action patterns.

That is, you might try the 'one-after-another-approach' that Patrick MacDonald describes, addressing the primary control from the 'top down', one part after another, and then out to the extremities and then, having all that organized to the best of your ability, piece together the action in a step-by-step manner.

And perhaps try the approach suggested in the 'Applications' section, analysing the action pattern into its elemental movements and, addressing the primary control in an 'all-at-once' fashion, then try the action as a combination of its elements.

In a last exploration, taking what may be a more 'internalized' and fluid approach, experiment with the sense and action of the soma releasing upwards from the ground and expanding out of the centre via a detailed address to the head-neck-spine-trunk-core; attending to the leading parts of the movement; to the connectedness of the somatic self in the action from top to bottom, centre to periphery, and fingers to toes, and through the central axis; to the body as a whole, epitomized in the centre of gravity, moving through the action in a flowing manner; looking for a minimization of effort, using the potential energy of 'radically upright' acture to initiate the 'power' of the movement and allowing the larger muscles to do the larger work and the smaller muscles the smaller work; and seeking a fullness and evenness in the cycling of the breathing.

In experimenting with these three approaches over time you may find that one or another is most useful for you in improving the quality of your action.

We will see with Awareness Through Movement another approach to piecing together an action pattern.

While the Technique is, in principle, about the way and not the goal, function will tend to improve as self-organization improves. From any 'normal' patterning, in general, as self-organization improves, the head will revolve forward and up from the top of the spine, the spine lengthen, the arms via the shoulder girdle release apart, the shoulders and back broaden, the hips release apart, the legs release out of the back via the pelvis, the frontal line open and lengthen and the ribcage come up. In a person who is hyperextended in the bodily pattern of effort or due to an unusual trauma or for some other reason such as a whiplash, the changes will be essentially the same but may appear differently.

AWARENESS THROUGH
MOVEMENT

To gain further agility, adaptability and grace in movement, of great value are Moshe Feldenkrais' Awareness Through Movement lessons (or ATM). Awareness Through Movement is an effective means of learning, through self-study in the context of designed movement sequences, what might be called 'unconscious constructive control' of oneself in action.

Where the context of the Alexander Technique, in its address to the primary control of action in the actural dynamic, is the exploration of the response to gravity that supports all movement, Awareness Through Movement is the exploration of movement itself and the concomitant improvement of sensory self-awareness. Where the Technique is more about buoyancy ATM is more about flow.

Feldenkrais was a physicist, master judoka, Gurdjieffian and educator. After a debilitating knee injury where the recommended surgery offered a doubtful success he undertook an in-depth investigation of his movement capabilities and eventually of human movement in general. In that process he not only regained his own ability to walk but also developed a technology of human movement and a method for refining the quality of movement through enhancing self-awareness that has found wide-ranging applications.

The Feldenkrais Method, which grew from his decades-long study, is a complex and evolving system integrating neuroscience and the movement sciences. The Method uses sophisticated manipulations to facilitate alternative patterns of action that are increasingly harmonious with the individual's structure and better adapted to the mechanical requirements of the surrounding world. These manipulations are founded in an understanding of human psychomotor development and function and of the systemic nature of function.

The Feldenkrais Method is a form of somatic education founded on the huge adaptability or learning capacity of the nervous system. In this method the sensorimotor cortex and nervous system are understood as a conjoint somatic process that mediates intelligence and organizes the individual's response to experience. The understanding that learning depends on the unconscious processes of the nervous system is made explicit in the Feldenkrais Method.

The Method has two lesson forms: Awareness Through Movement, verbally guided work, and Functional Integration® (FI®), hands-on one-on-one work. Awareness Through Movement lessons are technical designed movement explorations in which the teacher verbally guides students through a coherent series of developmental, biomechanical or functional movement patterns (for example, flexion, extension, reaching, turning, rolling, crawling or elaborations resembling complex acrobatic sequences), draws attention to the sensations elicited by these movements, and thereby facilitates, in an intriguing manner, improved coordination and a widening self-awareness. The lessons are interesting, refreshing and relaxing. They increase flexibility and suppleness without strain; improve efficiency while reducing effort; and can, over time, free the individual from chronic or acute pain. Because ATMs take ingenious advantage of the virtually unlimited learning potential of the human nervous system, anyone can improve his or her movement capabilities and, through practice, this improvement can be continuous. During training, Feldenkrais once said, in a quote that has passed into Feldenkrais lore, that through this work 'the impossible becomes feasible, the feasible becomes easy, the easy comfortable, enjoyable and aesthetically satisfying. That means learning.'

A Functional Integration lesson is a hands-on process, tailored to an individual's presenting limitations. Using refined touch and skilful handling, the practitioner gains an intelligent sense of the person's unique neuromotor patterning, and thereby initiates, stimulates and constructs a process of sensorimotor learning, clarifying and then undoing patterns of habitual tension and stereotyped movement and leading the person to better coordination options. Typically the practitioner moves the client who is passive. The practitioner seeks to duplicate or mirror the client's habitual patterning. By thus sensitively reflecting to the client his or her own patterning, the practitioner enables the person to become aware of, and thereby think and feel through, the patterns that limit the quality of movement. This growing awareness is the foundation of coming to sense oneself better and thus to move better. The effects of these lessons range from improvement in well-being and vitality, ease and efficiency to alleviation of pain and enhanced performance. Like ATMs, FIs are founded in the understanding that a person changes most readily when the newly proposed means of action are more pleasant than the old, that effectiveness comes through reducing effort – by working 'smarter' not harder – and that learning is natural and pleasurable.

Like the Technique, the Feldenkrais Method in general and ATM in particular use the mental faculties of attention, intelligence and intention, though less explicitly.

Because most ATMs are done in variations of sitting or lying on the ground, the importance of the primary control as the organization and organizer of movement in the actural dynamic is minimized. The requirement of the muscles that would otherwise be occupied with our upright response to gravity is virtually eliminated, thereby increasing the availability of attention to the parts and the movement of the parts – a use of the Weber–Fechner principle.

Some ATMs are designed as developmental learning patterns, re-establishing the ground for good use in the upright state.

Intention appears in the form of 'constraints' (verbal and bio-mechanical) and in the pupil following the directions called for. Intelligence lies in the device that is the design of the lesson itself and the manner in which it is to be carried out. In addition, intelligence of the participant is called for in his or her growing understanding of the principles of good movement, which principles are often iterated as meta-commentary through the lesson.

The movement sequences can be framed as a connected series of positive and negative constraints – what to do and how and what not to do and how not. The student is called to attend to the sensory and perceptual effects stimulated by the movement sequences. As these are noticed, that information is clarified, thereby enhancing sensory appreciation, which in turn improves the quality of movement, which improvement can potentially be transferred from floor movements to functioning in the actural dynamic. This process also somewhat duplicates infantile development, from prolonged play on the floor to the readiness for walking and standing.

Moreover, each lesson is designed to effect improved coordination of a functional pattern: from simple patterns such as reaching, rolling and so on to complex manoeuvres that can only be grasped when done.

Our individual patterning has a complex of causes dependent upon our histories. ATMs are processes of self-exploration *in relation to* our individual patterning and *in the context of* designed functional, biomechanical or developmental movement sequences through which that patterning can be uncovered and resolved. The manner in which movements are explored is generally via analysis and synthesis: the breaking down of the movement into its elemental parts and the performance of those parts, followed by the putting together of the parts.

ATMs are elemental human movements from which functional movements in daily life are developed. Like work in the Alexander Technique they are practiced as exercises of self-exploration and of attention not as exercises of the muscles.

They are typically 'groundwork' because by reducing the requirements of responding to gravity in the actual dynamic certain benefits ensue: the immense whole-body response of the anti-gravity mechanisms is virtually eliminated, thereby reducing the amount of input to the sensory nervous system and indirectly increasing the degree of sensitivity to kinaesthetic information. Thus, the person can more easily sense how to do the movement called for and how he or she is approximating that movement.

ATMs are also typically groundwork because of the additional feedback about our organization provided through the tactile sense by contact with the floor. This feedback that is extra to kinaesthesia is called redundant and is a feature of our common experience whereby the nervous system compares and correlates the information from a variety of senses in order to come to a congruent perception. It was the essence of Alexander's strategy of observing himself in mirrors – to give himself information from a dependable sense, vision – to calibrate and corroborate or correct his kinaesthesia.

ATMs' novelty arouse curiosity through their interesting designs. They stimulate a refining of awareness through the movements' stimulation of changes in the information to the senses. In expanding and correlating the sensory feedback, movement becomes more refined, which further refines the quality of self-sensing. Patterns that interfere with the best use of the self are clarified and resolved.

In *Constructive Conscious Control of the Individual*, Alexander suggested that, to improve the quality of any action pattern, one break the proposed action into parts and then put those parts together in sequence while maintaining good use. This is the essence of ATM. Where Alexander's description suggests a linear approach ATMs are generally anything but linear.

When Feldenkrais was living in London and developing his method he began lessons with Walter Carrington in the offices where Alexander taught and ran his training school. The story goes that one day Feldenkrais left a draft of his new book, *Body and Mature Behaviour*, for Alexander to peruse. When Alexander discovered that his own great contribution to the somatic field was unacknowledged he was indignant. He asked Carrington to 'cease and desist' teaching Feldenkrais who consequently continued lessons with a student of Alexander's first training, Charles Neale. It may be that Feldenkrais' pointed criticism in *Body and Mature Behaviour* (1950) of what he described as 'the overuse of the conscious control' contributed to Alexander's irritation. Alexander may also have reacted to Feldenkrais' ideas in that they made explicit, via the latter's explication of the self-organizing capability of the nervous system, the understanding that Alexander had been using implicitly but lacked the science to justify. During the first training course Lulie Westfeldt (1998) reports that one day Alexander entered class with the pronouncement, 'Now I can get it in spite of them' – meaning, I gather, that he had developed his handling to such a level of refinement that he could bypass the pupil's conscious control and could thereby inform the sensorimotor nervous system directly. In addition, where Alexander spoke of 'the sending of energies' via direction to the parts of the body to rightly organize the primary control, Feldenkrais may have appeared, by giving the psychophysical event a seemingly scientific neurological explanation, to provide that process of 'sending of energies' a more convincing foundation, which Alexander seems to have been seeking. Much of the neurophysiological data in Feldenkrais' book has since proved incomplete. Neuroscience continues to investigate the nervous system's role in sensorimotor functioning. Hypotheses have become very sophisticated and they are bound forever to prove incomplete. From the point of view of the soma and the refining of somatic competence a so-called objective explanation is inconsequential because somatic experience is not merely objective. In the 1970s Adi Da Samraj wrote, 'Watch for it. The nervous system will become the new golden calf' (Samraj 1977). This is, in fact, what has happened. Alexander's self-study was scientific and somatic, not objective, and it is unfortunate if he felt the need for objective support for his discoveries. His discoveries are self-authenticating and do not require justification or validation by objective explanations, no matter how sophisticated. In any case, your somatic experience is not in or of the nervous system but in and of the 'true water' of consciousness.

AN ANALYSIS OF MOVEMENT

Coordinating any movement sequence may be more easily accomplished with an understanding of the components of movement, which, by bringing into the foreground fundamental motor concepts, allows for a means whereby the organization of any movement may be accurately assessed and assembled.

Larry Goldfarb, a senior Feldenkrais practitioner, has developed a model that he calls SPIFFER whereby any action sequence can be analyzed into a family of motor concepts. The acronym refers to: Sequence, Path, Initiation, Flow, Foundation, Effort and Respiration. Using this model, an action pattern 'cascades' sequentially through the skeleton; the body's centre of mass follows a path through space; a part initiates the movement; the movement has a measure of smoothness or flow; it has a ground or foundation; there is some effort (in the physical sense of the term) involved; and we are breathing or respiring well or poorly. The bony aspect of the skeleton that moves first defines the initiation of the movement. In the view of the Alexander Technique, the head moves first in its release from the top of the central axis followed by the back to its base. From that prior coordination, the hand may go forward in reaching or gesturing or grasping or the knee forward in walking and so on. As any action pattern extends through a moment of time, the body as a linked structure goes through a sequence of changes in shape moment to moment as the centre of gravity follows a path through space. The foundation of any movement is the base of support of the movement, which, in the actural dynamic, is usually under the feet or sitting bones. The effort is the totality of muscular activity, whether synergistic or parasitic, helping or hindering. The measure of flow is determined by the degree of harmony of that muscular activity and how the force is coordinated through the body as a combined compression-tensegrity structure. By understanding that effort is best employed by the central muscles doing the greater work, the peripheral muscles doing the refined work, one can generate a more effective and flowing action. Respiration is disturbed if the effort is not harmonious.

By understanding any action sequence, in ATM or in daily life, in terms of this family of motor concepts one can nicely judge and thereby calibrate the quality of any present movement.

The purpose of ATM is to improve the quality of movement and self-sensing. You can assess the quality of your movements, using the SPIFFER model as a guide, by the measure of coordinated effort, alignment with the direction of force, freedom of breathing, and the clarity of the movement's foundation and its initiation, of its connectedness through the skeleton, and the measure of flow in the body's path through space.

The movements in an ATM lesson themselves do not have an obvious goal, so end-gaining is obviated by the apparent purposelessness of the movements and by the call for attention to the quality of the movement being explored. Goals emerge through the design of the lesson. It is the organization of the movement and the sensory body to which one pays attention and to the self-perceptions synthesized by the nervous system.

For instance, consider an instruction such as, 'Reach your arm towards the ceiling.' It is the sensations elicited by the movement and the organization of the movement that are the essence of the instruction, not the ceiling or the extent of the reach. Intentionally attending to the organization and quality of the movement obviously facilitates the ability to pay attention. Refining attention refines movement.

Each movement is generally repeated many times. The repetition allows you to study the movement in detail, feel it and yourself more and better each time, thereby improving the quality of your coordination and movement. Repetition is not useful if it is rote. Repetition is to enhance clarity and smoothness and to stimulate learning.

Doing the movement slowly enough that you can pay attention is also vital. Doing the movements slowly reduces the sensory input to the muscle spindles and thereby makes attention to the movements easier as per the Weber–Fechner principle. Moving quickly, brusquely or in a strained or stressed manner or in order to get a result of any kind distracts attention from the movement itself and thereby diminishes the potential for refining sensorimotor competence.

You always do less than you can because, when you do less than you know that you can, you know you can always do more. This relaxes efforting. Doing less allows the improvement to emerge on its own because improvement of function is spontaneous when one is observant and curious. Doing less than you can decreases sensory stimulation so that you are less distracted by your own work. This increases your ability to sense movement in a more refined and detailed manner. As sensory awareness becomes more differentiated and subtle, so movement becomes more differentiated and subtle. When you are doing less than you can, you are shifting your attention from any projected goal of the movement to the movement itself. When you do less than you can, your nervous system familiarizes itself with the direction and manner of the movement and in thus putting together how the movement is organized in and as the bodily self, improvement of movement quality and complexity naturally develops, as walking develops from infantile self-explorations. When you do less than you can you are also minimizing excessive muscular contracting.

In ATM, you want the movements to feel pleasant because pleasant sensations are enjoyable and as your ability improves through such enjoyable self-exploration, you will want to continue to improve your ability. When you do what is not pleasant, even if the results seem to represent an improvement, you will not naturally choose to do it and, without the ongoing effort of misplaced willpower, you may tend to give it up. New possibilities are better accepted as viable options when pleasant. Thus, willpower, trying harder and trying to get a result are devalued as means for learning in the Feldenkrais Method because they don't work. Rather, results develop naturally from the Method's technology and from the self-organizing capability of the nervous system.

PAIN AS MISINFORMATION

In ATMs (and yoga), feedback from the sensory realm in terms of pain should guide practice and, in that sense, all ATMs and asanas are to be approached with sensitivity. When an action or pose is merely uncomfortable one can use that discomfort as information to be understood. It is then like other kinaesthetic information, a sensation that can improve self-sensing, coordination and movement. When pain is great the nervous system responds reflexively by splinting the area around the pain. Actions that stimulate such pain and reflexive reaction should be avoided.

It is useless to 'push through the pain' aggressively or because it is deemed effective to go further and gain a greater result – because it is not effective to the end of improving function or awareness. It tends rather to limit functional improvements by stimulating a reflexive reaction, immobilizing a part of oneself in reaction to the pain in the moment or after the pushing through; and it undermines awareness because the pain 'speaks so loudly' that other sensory information is barred from registering, even especially the sensory information that one is immobilizing or contracting the musculature in the area of the pain.

Complete reliance on the self-organizing capability of the nervous system in its preference for what is pleasurable is not generally a sufficient practice. Because attention wanders to that to which it habitually wanders and poor habits of action tend to follow, the results of which are often limiting, unpleasant, distressing or painful, something else is required. Thus, the present-time (and at least random) coupling of attention with intelligence and intention serves to reinforce learning. This is the thesis with respect to the universal constant of use.

ATMs rely on 'doing and feeling', that is, one moves oneself and attends to the sensory effects of the movement. One's attention is to be directed 'outwards' to the doing of any action and at the same time 'inwards' to the organization and ongoing sensory effects of the action. Where there is a binding pattern or constricted tissue one can neither move nor feel competently. Constraints and variations help to overcome this limitation.

The principles of good movement, when kept in mind or taught as meta-commentary, are also helpful, the idea being that the principles will be spontaneously applied.

Generally, binding patterns are not suspected unless there is a sense of failure, limitation or pain. Even then, the actual source or nature of the bondage is not readily uncovered. Alexander's investigation revealed that, in the case of a functional limitation, there is always misuse of the primary control, a retraction of the head and a contraction in towards the centre and down via the central axis. The pattern is general but the idiosyncrasies of that patterning are unique to each person. The primary control as a motor concept represents a feed-forward image against which the distortions of form and function may be compared. Failure, conflict, pain and limitation tend to come after, even long after, the repetition of a poor habit pattern whereas disorganization of the primary control is the present 'cause' of the faulty pattern.

It is important to work with many ATMs as a means of resolving shortcomings. Variety is one of the very strategies for substantive improvement. Variety serves to reveal and more and more unravel the patterns of disorganized function through many takes on one's patterning. Variety serves to overcome state-specific learning. The hundreds of ATMs invented by Feldenkrais provide an enormous variety of sensorimotor experiences.

ATMs coax out new possibilities through verbal and mechanical constraints. A verbal constraint obliges you to do a movement in a particular way; a mechanical constraint requires you to work out a movement while restricted by a particular coordination or position or by the floor. The movement thus evoked, however small, can provide a new perception if the movement is large enough to cross the threshold of sensibility. A new perception can provide a building block for clearer self-sensing and thus, improved movement possibilities and so, with the addition of sufficient numbers of such new possibilities, the indirect bypassing and resolution of binding patterns.

The keys to benefiting from ATM practice are the quality of one's attention; the precision and the biomechanical integration with which one carries out the movements; the variety in timing and of positions and orientations in which one does the movement and its variations; the range within which one can comfortably carry out the movements; the integration into a larger 'bodily self-image' of the many sensations elicited; and the application of the principles of good movement to the exercise.

A typical ATM follows a developmental, biomechanical or functional theme at the end of which new possibilities emerge. The goals of an ATM are multifold: they may include that emergent movement, an improvement in the so-called reference movement that sometimes begins a lesson, the variety of means, improved general function or greater awareness. Even the manner of learning can be considered part of the purpose of a lesson.

A model ATM lesson or lesson series will address a pattern that is global or local, bilateral or unilateral. That pattern is analyzed into its elemental functional components whose performance stimulates a variety of sensory experiences. These experiences effect a re-calibration of the movement, an emergent learning – what Alexander called a 'going into the unknown'. This learning is reinforced by repetition or exploration of the functional changes in various orientations, rhythms and degrees. The thus improved quality of movement obviates limitations by mastering an action pattern.

The functional changes induced by an ATM should be reinforced at the end of the lesson. The fact and force of sensorimotor unreliability and habit must be understood. The student, rising into the upright state at the end of a lesson, is often met with many new sensations, which may seem paramount. Because each person has individual limitations and because each ATM, as an address to a general pattern, therefore affects each person differently, the sensory results of the lesson manifest differently in each of us and thus cannot always be addressed by a general admonition or instruction. As Alexander determined, these unfamiliar sensory and perceptual effects should be largely ignored as they tend to be unreliable. The motor changes are more significant and reliable. By exploring in the actural dynamic the movement and coordination changes realized in the lesson while at the same time reflecting on the perceivable changes in the organization of the self *vis-à-vis* the primary control, the sensory peculiarities become less distracting and disappear over time.

Most ATMs are performed in some orientation that reduces the effects of responding to gravity so that the sensory load is reduced, the habits associated with the upright state are avoided and the ability to pay attention thereby indirectly increased. In ATMs you are working on patterns within the whole. It is important, in the return to the actural dynamic, to integrate the improvements that have emerged from the ATM by exploring related patterns in the new orientation. This exploration serves to integrate those changes such that the previously binding effects in the use of the parts are minimized and the improvement reinforced and integrated as a viable future option. As in an Alexander lesson, work lying down is followed by work again in the actural dynamic to integrate the changes wrought in the table work.

Where in the Alexander Technique the faculties are applied in direct service, so to speak, to the primary control, in Awareness Through Movement practice they are used more generally.

Awareness Through Movement consists of a network of interactive strategies that are the practical foundation of every lesson and are so interwoven that it is impossible to separate them in fact.

INTELLIGENCE

Play, curiosity and self-exploration are valued in ATM because they are effective, even necessary, learning strategies and also because the Method is in part a developmental learning model.

The enormous variety of Awareness Through Movement lessons, and so of sensorimotor experiences, is itself a means whereby new options are synthesized by the nervous system. Like a child's exploratory play, the sheer variety of experiences affords the nervous system multifaceted material, which makes for integration of function, enhanced self-sensing and improved movement. Unlike a child's play, the technical design of ATMs, which design brings the manipulation of movement to the level of a technology, eliminates much of the trial and error and randomness of childhood play and speeds the recovery of sensorimotor competence.

Intelligence lies in the complex technology of each lesson and in the student's use of the principles of good movement in feeling and thinking through each movement.

AWARENESS

The principal means of increasing functional self-awareness is through shifting attention from outward to inward. Often in our daily lives we are oriented to getting results in the outer world. The approach in ATM counters that tendency by recalling attention from gaining an end to the quality and the present-time organization and sensory effects of the action performed.

Attention to the breath and its congruence with the action is of vital importance as well.

Basic to the Method is the Weber–Fechner principle of smallest noticeable differences. Thus, a fundamental strategy is to minimize the stimuli so that smaller and smaller differences can be distinguished.

Lying on the floor removes the vast number of stimuli to the balance, pressure, tension and joint capsule receptors stimulated by the response to gravity in the upright state.

Moving slowly reduces the stimulation to the movement receptors. Moving more and more smoothly reduces confusing sensations to the movement receptors. Moving within the range of ease reduces stimulation of the pain receptors so that subtler feelings of discomfort can be discriminated or eliminated and appropriate tension, balance and force through the structure can be more easily sensed and calibrated.

Scanning of the body brings attention to proprioceptive and tactile data. In scanning, one feels oneself from the inside and uses the contact with the floor on the outside as further information.

Previous positions or movements are repeatedly revisited in order to compare one's present-time sense and organization of the position or movement with previous trials. This comparing or noticing of changes is a key to refining self-awareness.

Repetition of movements is for exploring and comparing and for improving awareness. Repetition is necessary because the movement must be repeated to get the maximum information from it. Repeating the movements with variations in timing and orientation enhances awareness and learning. Repetition is also for the purpose of refining the quality or 'intelligence' of the movement itself, which further refines the ability to sense clearly.

Interest is vital. The novelty of the movements performed in ATM is one of the very means to stimulate interest and awareness.

RELEASE AND DIFFERENTIATION

Release from binding patterning is a basic aim in any somatic learning method.

In ATM common strategies are: letting go parasitical contraction patterns; minimizing effort used; differentiating, in terms of both sensations and movements, the parts of the body from each other — say, the arm from the trunk or the pelvis from the lumbar spine; and exploring cardinal directions, circles or figures within a position or pattern. Letting go may also be found at the apparent end-range of a movement where one may simply be unaware that the movement can easily go further.

When a muscle is contracting, the antagonistic musculature is reciprocally inhibited. Thus every muscular contraction effects an inhibition of the antagonistic musculature. Attending to the lengthening musculature reinforces such release. Paradoxically, consciously contracting a muscle allows its better release because conscious control and release are functionally inextricable.

Rhythmic oscillations may be used to relax holding. When one sets up a rocking movement, typically with the feet or the pelvis, leaving the rest of the body to be involved passively in the oscillation, release within the pattern may be elicited and then use of the musculature within the pattern or position can be more readily achieved.

Paying attention to and bypassing any interruption of the breathing and manipulating the breath cycle are strategies used to resolve limitations in any pattern being explored.

A trick that may be tried in order to encourage the participation of a part in any movement is to fix that part to a part that moves easily and then move the latter part. For instance, if the neck is not participating or is uncomfortable in a movement, one might fix an extended arm to the head at the ear and then gently move the arm in circles with the head 'attached'. You might do this gently using the other arm or both arms and in various orientations. Doing this slowly and smoothly may allow the neck's participation in further explorations.

In addition, fixing the arm to the head constrains the movement of the neck, which encourages movement in the thoracic spine and ribs. Thus, the person may learn that, when moving the head, the thoracic vertebrae and ribs, and perhaps even the pelvis, can be involved and thus take the strain from the neck. Such temporary release can give one confidence that the limitation is not structural for its easy disappearance would not be possible given a structural basis, that the problem is therefore functional and resolvable with improved functioning.

Sometimes it seems impossible to work out a movement. Yet, most movements can be described as the articulation of one part of the body with another. If one is reaching an arm, say, then the arm is moving with respect to the trunk. If there seems to be a restriction in the movement being explored that cannot be overcome by trying to do it directly, a relative conjugate movement may be tried.

A relative conjugate movement moves the proximal part relative to the peripheral part: in the above case, the trunk relative to the arm instead of the arm relative to the trunk. This can induce the system into realizing the alternate pattern.

Thomas Hanna discovered an effective technique called pandiculation for releasing chronic muscle contraction, which he used explicitly in some of his 'somatic exercises' and in his hands-on work. Pandiculations are used implicitly in some ATMs though it is not clear that Feldenkrais knew the neuromuscular basis of the process. A pandiculation is a deliberate strong voluntary muscle contraction followed by its slow controlled release.

Your morning 'stretch' is, in fact, a whole-body pandiculation that, as such, reawakens the musculature and quickens its return to voluntary control. Through the strong controlled contraction and de-contraction (or eccentric contraction) of a muscle a pandiculation provides clear sensory information relative to the use of that muscle to the nervous system. Typically in an ATM, it is gravity as it affects the position in which one is working that provides the force against which one is contracting. For instance, lying prone and extending (arching) the trunk requires working against the push of gravity. If you raise the head and arms and legs slowly and smoothly and return to the prone position similarly, you are pandiculating the extensor musculature of the back and legs and arms.

If an ATM is one that is designed to improve the lengthening of the back, then a pandiculation might be used as in the above example. The slow strong contraction of the extensor musculature and the slowness of the release deliver a large amount of information in terms of the use of that musculature to the sensory cortex and enforce attention to the means whereby one is using that musculature, eliciting thereby a cortical override of the subcortical pattern. With each pandiculation the 'normal' tone may release and more and more with each application. The new 'normal' may then be reinforced through reciprocal inhibition, by touching or tapping the musculature released to bring awareness to the musculature or by an exploratory movement in the context of the pattern. Pandiculation is both a neurological and a somatic event.

In a system that is 'shouting loudly' with chronic pain or contraction patterns, the call in ATM to move gently, while frequently necessary, sometimes suffers the limitation that a small new stimulus may not be registered or deemed 'useful' by the nervous system. The idea that lying down can quiet every system such that subtle manipulations can be 'heard' is not always tenable. The subtle input offered in a typical Alexander or Feldenkrais lesson will sometimes not be sufficient. The Weber–Fechner principle suggests that a proportionately larger stimulus may be given.

It is sometimes only in the repetition of experiences in these cases that the system eventually 'hears'. That is why it is not unknown for a pupil to say, after several weeks of lessons, something like, 'We've never done that before,' when that manipulation or movement has been repeated many times in the course of lessons. Only by then, enough change has occurred in the person that the movement is noticed for the first time.

Quieting the system is not always accomplished by the typical means. What can sometimes succeed is to speak 'loudly' and well enough that the system can hear over its own self-generated noise. This is the reason, I think, that my first teacher needed to be so firm at the start of my training. Pandiculation and deep monkey, when well-organized, can provide this 'loud' information as can the powerful coordinated contractions in some yoga poses. A few of the ATMs Feldenkrais recorded at his studio in Tel Aviv seem to address this issue though he did not indicate the neurophysiological reasons behind his use of the more affirmative functional demands in these lessons.

DIRECTED MOVEMENT

As one senior Feldenkrais trainer has quipped, 'Language is the organization of the organization of action.' This was Alexander's practice in giving himself verbal directions in order to facilitate better organization of his actions. An ATM is a series of instructions that are designed to organize the pupil's action through a coordination of congruent movements. These instructions make for a complex of constraints, verbal and mechanical.

An instruction obliges you to do what you sometimes cannot do immediately, can only do minimally or cannot do well. Because every movement called for is composed of elements of movements learned in the past, one can generally accomplish a first approximation. Repeated experimental trials are often then the key to learning. It is psychologically important to reframe so-called 'trials and errors' as 'trials and partial successes' to bypass the association of practice with failure.

Two basic principles of the Method are: there are no rules in an exploration and if what you're doing isn't working, try something else.

Sometimes there seems to be no way to accomplish the action suggested. It may then be useful to analyze the movement into even more manageable pieces or from different orientations and then put the whole movement back together. Sometimes it can be effective to use imagination. Such imagining has been proven to effect neuromotor changes, minutely activating the very musculature involved in accomplishing the action in reality. When the musculature is thus minutely used, movements within the threshold of sensation may then be tried.

Another strategy is to do the movement badly. This undermines the psychological compulsion to get it right and also affords a means of comparing the actual action done poorly with the imagined action done well – that is, smoothly, with uninterrupted breathing, with skeletal connectedness, a clear foundation and leading parts and with appropriate tone and a coordinated effort – which the nervous system reads similarly. By inventing errors, one can come to a better means of approximating the movement called for through comparing the poorly accomplished movement with the more accurately conceived movement.

A technique used in some lessons is to work with the easy side or the easier unilateral pattern first. Feldenkrais discovered that information from one side of the sensorimotor cortex transfers readily to the other side via the corpus callosum. Thus, in refining the quality of movement on the easier side first, the movement is then more easily accomplished on the less agile side. Having done the movement on the one side, the related sensations and the movements are already familiar and therefore one can look and allow for similar sensorimotor events on the second side. This makes learning quicker on the second side and potentially then, the motor accomplishments can be taken beyond their expected limit as a result.

One is never to go beyond what is comfortable so that there is no association of distress with the process of learning. By staying within what is comfortable one is called to do the mere movement. Whether one does the movement to its limit or stays within a pleasurable range the organization of the musculature is essentially the same. This coordination or means whereby of the movement is what is to be learned and is what accomplishes the movements. Therefore, by staying within the range of what is easy, the movement becomes easier and the range will naturally increase because greater freedom, competence and comfort are sought by the nervous system.

EMERGENT LEARNING

It is implied in some new-age thinking that, with improvements in sensorimotor function, improvements emerge in psychological and emotional patterning. This has not been corroborated by evidence. To believe that integrating the function of the pelvis, for instance, into the global pattern of movement will resolve a person's concomitant complication with respect to matters 'below the belt' is a belief that may rest on a belief that the cerebral cortex governs rather than mediates cognition and feeling, that the soma is an epiphenomenon of the brain, or that thinking, feeling, sensing and moving are a 'democracy' not a hierarchy of functions. Emotions and thinking are expressed or suppressed somatically. Thought moves the vocal organs subtly for instance; emotion changes the breath. Becoming sensitive enough to notice such things may allow one to relax the parasitical pattern.

A Zen roshi apparently commented to Patrick MacDonald that mastering the Alexander Technique would eliminate twenty years of sitting practice. While probably spoken in hyperbolic terms, this may have some truth because the body reflects, indeed embodies, either through expression or suppression, the self-contracted processes and states of mind and emotion and because practice can relax such physical reactivity. Releasing the body from its patterns towards its natural state may serve to uncover or weaken habitual emotional and mental states and processes. Freud observed that psychological patterning is over-determined and that no analysis can be complete. Release of patterning may be made direct in this work and may thus prepare one for the gesture beyond mind in the Zen sense.

INTEGRATION

The fundamental purposes of ATM are functional integration – all the parts, from fingers to toes and head to tail participating harmoniously and congruently in any action pattern – sensorimotor learning and 'unconscious constructive control' of the self in action. Awareness, intelligence, release and directed action together serve these ends. Indeed, awareness cannot be separated from integration as sensing cannot be separated from movement and the organization of movement. Still, there are distinct strategies that serve integration more than anything else.

One of these is the designed result of each lesson. Each lesson is intended to accomplish and integrate an action pattern. Many lessons serve to promote greater symmetry. Improved symmetry, both in terms of motor ability and in terms of sensory balance, is a sign of integration and is often important for competent function.

The Method is founded on the self-organizing capability of the nervous system: given a chaos of information, the nervous system will select and order the information to fulfill its needs. This capability realizes the emergent learning that is the effect of every lesson. Many lessons or lesson series are designed to review some small part of infantile or childhood development, the results of which in each of us would have been more competent adaptation to adult function.

Thus, the emergent learning can be a renewal, recapitulation, elaboration, refinement or approximation of a developmental learning. Another means used is resting. By resting after a period of exploration, the nervous system assimilates, processes and reorganizes the sensorimotor information. Often after a rest a movement that was difficult or inefficient becomes remarkably clearer and easier.

Returning to earlier movements in the sequence integrates and confirms the changes. Moreover, in going back to those movements as the lesson progresses, one will find that one is both sensing more of oneself and allowing more parts of the body to participate synergistically in the movement. This synergism in the coordination of the movement and this sensing of more of the parts involved are further signs of integration of function.

Finally, the particular strategy of moving the eyes or the head congruently with or in opposition to the global or local movement being explored can elicit participation of the head and spinal axis of the body, which, as the core of the primary control, serves the integration of function.

INTELLIGENCE IN ACTION
ATM Series

ATM STRATEGIES

Intelligence

Playful attitude, curiosity, interest
Varieties of sensorimotor experience
SPIFFER

Awareness

Weber–Fechner/reducing 'noise'/slowness and smoothness
Scanning
Shifting of attention from outer to inner
Repetition as exploration

Release/differentiation

Minimizing effort and parasitical contractions
Exploration of circles within the pattern
Manipulation of breathing
Relative conjugate movements
Reciprocal inhibition/lengthening antagonistic musculature
Pandiculation

Directed movement

Constraints
Working with easy side first and comparing differences
Breaking down the movement into manageable pieces

Making things worse/inventing errors
Imagining movement

Integration
Noticing/allowing synergistic movements
Variations in speed, rhythm, size, position and orientation
Rests
Eye and head movements
Returning to earlier movements
Reinforcing/practicing emergent movements

In general, begin and end each ATM with a supine scan, a standing scan and a walking scan. At the end of the lesson check in the actrual dynamic any thematic elements. One should follow the sequences of lessons here, developing at least a basic understanding of and competence at one before proceeding to the next. Before attempting these ATMs attend classes for a while or work with online ATMs recorded by different practitioners (at www.openatm.org or www.kinesophics.ca) to get a working understanding of the approach.

Each instruction in the following ATMs is a guideline whose components you can break into more manageable pieces. Once you have some familiarity with the lessons you can, at the easy end-range of any movement, explore optional movements such as circles perpendicular to the direction of the movement, flexion and extension of the spine, turning of the head with or in opposition to the eyes, or breathing manipulations as described in the 'Ball of Air' ATM. You can do the movement in your imagination. You can think of ways of doing the movement badly. You can vary the speed, size, orientation or rhythm of the movement or also the focus of your attention. *That is, you may focus, during the progress of any movement, on the initiation, sequence, source of effort, foundation or changing shape of the movement or the centre of gravity's path through space or on any particular part of the body.* Repeatedly return to previous movements in the instructions to see that what you have done subsequently has improved the quality of a previous movement.

Each movement should be done slowly, even very slowly, and lightly and as accurately as possible many times, each time as an exploration and as many times as there continues to be interest, staying within the range of what is comfortable, only increasing the range of the movement as it becomes easy.

Look for a synergy of effort, a coordination and sequence of muscular effort and skeletal linkage from head to tail, head to toes, fingers to toes, and periphery to centre. (As the pelvis moves is the head responding? As the head moves is the pelvis following? As you reach with a leg, is there a response of an arm? As you reach with an arm is there a response in a leg?) Seek to leave the rhythm of the breathing undisturbed. *Each segment always involves the movement instructed and the return to the starting position of the movement with equal and global attention in both.* After a one-sided sequence compare the two sides in supine. *Always pause a few moments before performing the next movement and rest in supine for a minute or so after three or four sets of movements.* At the end of the lesson, register and explore, in supine, changes in the primary image and, in the actural dynamic, changes in the primary control and function.

SCANS

Supine scan

Lie supine and make yourself comfortable.

Give your attention to the contact of the body with the floor at the heels, calves, thighs, buttocks and through the buttocks the pelvis, tailbone and sacrum, the ribcage, the parts of the shoulders and arms and hands, and the head.

Compare the two sides in terms of the degrees and sizes of the areas of contact at the heels, calves, thighs, buttocks, pelvis, sacrum, ribcage, shoulders, arms, hands and sides of the head.

Now bring your attention to inner sensations: the angles of the joints: the ankles, knees, hips, the curves of the spine, the shoulders, elbows, wrists, fingers and the curve of the neck; sensations of compression, perhaps in the lumbar spine, neck or belly; sensations of tension, perhaps in the neck or the backs of the knees;

any feelings of discomfort, perhaps at points of contact with the floor or other areas that are chronic; feelings of inner space.

Compare the apparent length or shortness of the legs, the arms and the sides of the trunk. Compare the relative orientation of the feet and legs, arms and hands. Guess the shape of the spaces behind the knees, the small of the back, the shoulders, wrists and neck.

Does the pelvis seem shifted or rotated or hiked up or back? Does the ribcage seem shifted or rotated, pulled forward or lifted up, or pulled down to one side or the other? Does the head seem turned or shifted or pulled up or down or to one side or the other?

Does anything else stand out to your attention?

Observe these things freely.

Standing scan

For this you will need perhaps half a dozen firm foam kneeling pads. Stack two or three about four to six inches from a wall and stand preferably in firm-soled shoes such that the heels are against the wall, the balls of the feet are on the stack of pads and there is a very mild stretch on the calves and backs of the knees. If the head is not against the wall, place a few pads on the shoulders behind the head so that the head rests against the pads.

Relax in standing and make yourself comfortable.

Give your attention to the contact of the body with the wall at the heels, perhaps the calves, and the buttocks and through the buttocks perhaps the pelvis, tailbone and sacrum, the ribcage, parts of the shoulders and perhaps the arms and hands and the head.

Compare the two sides in terms of the degrees and sizes of the areas of contact both under and behind the heels, at the calves, buttocks, pelvis, sacrum, ribcage, shoulders, arms, hands and the sides of the head.

Now bring your attention to inner sensations and perceptions: the angles of the joints: the ankles, knees, hips, the curves of the spine, the shoulders, elbows, wrists, fingers and the curve of the neck; sensations of compression, perhaps in the lumbar spine, the neck or the belly, perhaps the knees or ankles, the shoulders or ribcage; sensations of tension or stretch, perhaps in the neck or the backs of the knees, the arms and shoulders; any feelings of discomfort that are chronic; feelings of inner space.

Compare the apparent length or shortening of the legs, arms and sides of the trunk. Compare the relative orientation of the two feet and the two legs, the two arms and two hands. Guess the shape of the spaces behind the legs, the small of the back, the arms and the neck.

Does the pelvis seem shifted or rotated or hiked up or back? Does the ribcage seem shifted or rotated, pulled forward or lifted up, or pulled down to one side or the other? Does the head seem turned or shifted or pulled back or forward or to one side or the other?

Notice any feelings of weight or compression through the frame that the standing pose makes evident. Observe the breathing and the effect that standing has on it. How does the bodily self-image in standing compare to that in supine?

Does anything else stand out to your attention?

Observe these things freely.

Variation: Interlace the fingers so that they are inside the palms. Place the hands on the crown of the head and relax the hands, arms and shoulders such that the weight of the arms pins the hands to the head and falls through the spine, pelvis and legs and into the floor, releasing the arms' weight from the ribcage. Observe any changes in the breathing.

Walking scan

For this, you will want a long hallway or sidewalk.

Walk easily, not measured, slowly or quickly. Relax the eyes.

Notice the heel strike and the passage of contact under the soles of the feet.

Notice the orientation of the feet and knees. Notice the swing of the legs.

Compare the feet, knees and legs.

Notice and compare the swing of the arms and directions and degrees of their swing.

Notice the carriage of the head.

Notice the movement of the pelvis. Do the hips move forward and back, in a rotation, and/or side to side?

Notice the carriage of the ribcage and the shoulders.

Does anything else stand out to your attention?

Observe these things freely.

ABBREVIATIONS

The following abbreviations will be used in the instructions:

S = supine, legs relaxed and lengthened out, arms relaxed and by the sides

SS = semi-supine

P = prone

SLL(R) = side-lying on the left (right) side, knees and hips at right angles

SL(R) = side-sitting left (right)

R(L)A = right (left) arm

R(L)E = right (left) elbow

R(L)L = right (left) leg

R(L)H = right (left) hand

R(L)K = right (left) knee

R(L)F = right (left) foot

H = head

SBR(L) = side-bend right (left)

PV = pelvis

RC = ribcage

HJ = hip joints

B = back

T = trunk

N = neck

BK = buttocks

ASIS = anterior superior iliac spine

PSIS = posterior superior iliac spine

→ and continue to

KNEE CIRCLES

Freeing the legs and hips, relaxing the lower back

Supine

Turn RF outward (right)

→ allowing RK, RL and PV to roll outward

→ allowing RK to bend, drawing RF towards BK, RK hanging outwards (= position #1 – that is, LL long, RL bent at knee with knee hanging outwards, RF in midline near BK)

From #1 bring RK to pointing to ceiling, RF standing flat on the floor in midline

Combine above movements from supine, turning RF outwards, RK, RL and PV rolling outward, drawing RF towards BK, RK hanging out, then bring RK to pointing at ceiling, RF standing

From #1 bring RK back and forth across midline, RF standing

From #1 bring RK across midline, RF standing and, with RK pointing medially, return RL to supine

Combine all movements, from supine, making clockwise circles with RK

Make counter-clockwise circles with RK

Repeat entire sequence with LL

Combine movements of LL and RL, making clockwise circles with RK and clockwise circles with LK, rolling onto left side

Combine movements of LL and RL, making counter-clockwise circles with RK and counter-clockwise circles with LK, rolling onto right side

ARM CIRCLES

Improving reaching

Side-lying left

Arms extended in front at shoulder height, palms together

Slide RH forward and back over LH

Slide RK forward and back over LK

Sweep RA at shoulder height in arc towards floor behind

Again, sweep RA in arc at shoulder height towards floor behind, pause near limit of range, and turn head back and forth

Point RA at ceiling, with LH move right shoulder blade back and forth on ribcage

Pointing RA at ceiling, reach RH towards ceiling and retract

Point RA at ceiling, reach RH towards ceiling while making screwing motion and retract with unscrewing motion

RH touching left ear over head, side-bend right, lifting feet and head

Turn head and shoulders to the right, interlace fingers behind the head and raise head and shoulders in twisted sit-up

Sweep RA in arc towards floor behind

Make (small and large, fast and slow) circles with RA in space

Reverse the direction of the circles

Repeat sequence with LA **side-lying right**

WASHRAG

Improving turning

Semi-supine

Steeple arms with fingers interlaced straight above the shoulders and tilt them right, then left, then side to side, rolling head with arms, then rolling head opposite to arms

With LH, pull straight RA via the wrist allowing the right shoulder blade to ease off the ribcage

With RH, pull straight LA via the wrist allowing the right shoulder blade ease off the ribcage

With soft fists, press RC everywhere

Cross legs, right thigh over left thigh, and tilt them right

Cross legs, left thigh over right thigh, and tilt them left

Cross legs, left thigh over right thigh, and tilt them left and pause, interlace fingers behind the head, and do twisted sit-ups

Cross legs, right thigh over left thigh, and tilt them right and pause, interlace fingers behind the head, and do twisted sit-ups

With legs glued together and arms steepled with fingers interlaced straight above the shoulders, take knees left as arms go right, and *vice versa*, turning head and eyes with arms

With legs glued together and arms steepled with fingers interlaced straight above the shoulders, take knees left as arms go right, and *vice versa*, turning head with knees and eyes with arms

PELVIC CLOCK

Freeing the pelvis

Semi-supine

Palpate borders of PV: pubic bone, inguinal ligaments, ASIS, iliac crest; sense back of PV on floor

Imagine you are lying on a clock face, the 12 o'clock towards L1, the 6 o'clock towards the tailbone, 3 o'clock towards PSIS on left, 9 o'clock towards PSIS on right

Rock PV towards 6; rock PV towards 12; combine movements

Rock PV towards 3; rock PV towards 9; combine movements

Rock PV around clock from 12 to 3, from 12 to 9, from 6 to 3, from 6 to 9, from 12 to 6 via 3, from 6 to 12 via 9

Make clockwise circles around clock; make counter-clockwise circles around clock

Rock PV from 1 to 7, from 2 to 8, from 3 to 9, from 4 to 10, from 5 to 11

Make clockwise, then counter-clockwise circles around the clock, make them larger/smaller, go slowly/quickly

Taking a wider stance let the knees fall together, and make clockwise and counter-clockwise circles, smaller, larger, faster, slower

Place RF on LK, RK pointing out, and make clockwise and counter-clockwise pelvic circles, smaller, larger, faster, slower

Place LF on RK, LK pointing out, and make clockwise and counter-clockwise pelvic circles, smaller, larger, faster, slower

FORWARD BENDING

Lengthening the back

Semi-supine

RH behind LK bent over RC, LH behind H, approximate LK and H

RH behind RK bent over RC, LH behind H, approximate RK and H

LH behind RK bent over RC, RH behind H, approximate RK and H

LH behind LK bent over RC, RH behind H, approximate LK and H

RH behind bent LK over RC, LH behind RK bent over RC, approximate H and feet

Leaning on elbows, pelvic clock

Leaning on hands, pelvic clock

Sitting with RL long, LF standing, H on LK, hands holding under LF, extend LL

Sitting with LL long, RF standing, H on RK, hands holding under RF, extend RL

Sitting, knees bent, feet standing, H on knees, hands holding under soles of feet, extend legs

Semi-supine

Sweep RA behind knees bent over RC, LH behind H, raise H and feet to ceiling

Sweep LA behind knees bent over RC, RH behind H, raise H and feet to ceiling

CAT AND COW

Integrating the axial skeleton

Sit on chair, round and arch the back, tailbone to crown

All fours, knees and hands shoulder width apart

Flex and extend the spine, tailbone to crown

Side-bend right and side-bend left, tailbone to crown

On knees and elbows, knees and elbows shoulder width apart

Flex and extend the spine, SBR and SBL

All fours, knees wider than hands

Flex and extend the spine, SBR and SBL

All fours, LK forward

Flex and extend the spine, SBR and SBL (same movements with RK forward)

Kneeling, RE on floor, LS on floor with LA through gap to the right between RK and RE, left side of H on floor, facing right

Flex and extend the spine, SBR and SBL (same movements with **body organized oppositely**)

All fours, with LF standing

Flex and extend the spine, SBR and SBL (same movements with **body organized oppositely**)

Standing on hands and feet, arms and legs extended

Flex and extend the spine, SBR and SBL

BALL OF AIR

Freeing the breath

Semi-supine (imagine the thoracic cavity divided into five sections: lower right and left, upper right and left, and a central section behind the xyphoid process)

Take a big breath and, holding that 'ball of air', push it slowly into the belly and then draw it slowly into the upper chest

Interlace the fingers behind H and flex and extend the back

Take a big breath and, holding the 'ball of air', push it slowly into the belly while flattening the back and pull the air slowly into the upper chest while arching the back

Interlace the fingers behind H, arch the back and, remaining in extension, take a big breath and slowly move the ball of air into the belly, into the centre, then into the upper chest

Interlace the fingers behind H, arch the back more, and take a big breath and slowly move the ball of air up and down

Side-lying right, left hand over H touching right ear, SBL take a big breath and slowly move the ball of air into the lower right section of the RC, then into the upper right

The **body arranged oppositely**, repeat the above instruction

Semi-supine

Take a big breath and slowly push the ball of air into the lower left, then through the central section into the upper right, then into the lower right, then through the centre into the upper left, then in circles

SILLY WALKING

Improving walking

Supine

Lay the LL at about 45° from the midline, stand the RF and, leaving the RK in the midline, straighten the RL by sliding the RF medially in an arc towards the LL

Lay the LL at about 45° from the midline, stand the RF and, leaving the RK in the midline, straighten the RL by sliding the RF laterally in an arc away from the LL

Combine the two movements, taking the RF in a circular movement while keeping the RK in the midline, standing and straightening the RL

Repeat the above movements with the LL

Make opposing circles with both feet while keeping the knees in the midline

Stand RF, tilt it left onto the inner edge of foot, and push with RF to roll the PV left, opening the RHJ and arching the back

→ extend the LA on floor above the head and continue the movement

→ turn H to look at LH and continue the movement

→ reaching with LA upwards as you continue the movement

→ reaching with RA towards RF as you continue the movement

Repeat the above movements, the **body arranged oppositely**, attending to the circular movements and opening and closing of the LHJ

Make opposing circles with both feet while keeping the knees in the midline

Lean back on extended arms and continue movement

TWISTING

Improving turning

Side-sitting left (sitting with knees bent and to the left, weight mostly on left buttock and thigh, RK against the sole of the LF, leaning to the left on left fist, RH on LS) **turned to left**

Pausing at the easy end-range of that turning, flex and extend the trunk, looking down in flexion and up in extension

Pausing at easy end-range of that turning, turn the head to the left and to the right

→ bend the neck looking down and arch the neck looking up

→ make circles with the nose

Turned left and keeping the eyes fixed on a point on the wall directly before you, flex and extend the trunk, bending the head down in flexion and up in extension

Turned left, turn the PV left, opening the RHJ and arching the back, then draw the PV back and down to the right, closing the RHJ and rounding the back

Turned left, turn the shoulder girdle to the left and to the right

Turned left, turn the shoulder girdle to the right while turning the PV to the left and then reverse those opposing movements

Turned left and fixing the eyes on a point directly before you, turn the head to the right while turning the trunk (shoulders and PV) to the left – and then reverse those opposing movements

Repeat the above sequence of movements with the **body arranged oppositely**

EXTENDING THE BACK

Lengthening the back

Prone, H turned right, LA by side, H on RH, RL frog-legged

Raise LL

Lift RE, H and RS together

Combine two movements

Repeat sequence, **the body arranged oppositely**

Semi-supine

LH behind RK bent over RC, RH behind LK bent over RC, approximate H and feet

Legs glued, tilt legs right and left

Prone, H turned R, fingers interlaced behind H, knees bent at 90°, soles of feet facing ceiling

Tilt legs left and right

Repeat above sequence, the **body arranged oppositely**

Semi-supine

Sweep LA behind knees bent over RC, raise H and feet to ceiling

Repeat above movement, the **body arranged oppositely**

Sitting, knees bent, feet standing, H on knees, hands holding undersoles of feet, extend legs

BACK ROLLER

Lengthening the back

(For this ATM, use a 3" thick, 3' long, hard foam roller or a very tightly rolled and bound blanket or beach towel)

Semi-supine with roller **vertically** along spine, arms extended to the side at shoulder height

Roll H left and right

Roll PV left and right

Roll PV and H oppositely

Tilt PV right turning H left as you roll RA at shoulder level and like a rolling pin down and LA at shoulder level and like a rolling pin up, then the reverse

Pelvic clock on roller, 12 o'clock to 6 o'clock

Supine on roller, flex and extend ankles, creating oscillations

Semi-supine, roller **horizontally** under sacrum, arms extended sideways at shoulder height

Extend legs, flex and extend ankles, creating oscillations

Glue bent legs together and tilt them left and right

Tilt legs right turning H left as you roll RA down and LA up, then the reverse

Hold RK over the RC with hands and make circles with the RK

Hold LK over the RC with hands and make circles with the LK

Sitting, knees bent, feet standing, H on knees, hands holding under soles of feet, extend legs

OPENING THE LEGS

Freeing the hip joints

Sitting with soles of the feet together leaning back on arms

Move the RF away from the LF

Move the LF away from the RF

Flex and extend the spine from the head to tail

Rotate the RF on its outer edge towards the toes, then the heel

Rotate the LF on its outer edge towards the toes, then the heel

Hold the RF in the hands, lift and make circles with it

Hold the LF in the hands, lift and make circles with it

Prone

With H facing right draw RK up into frog-legged position drawing right hip back and to the left

Repeat above movement with **body arranged oppositely**

Supine

Take hold of RK bent over RC with both hands and make clockwise, then counter-clockwise circles with the knee

Repeat above movement with **body arranged oppositely**

Sitting with soles of the feet together leaning back on extended arms

Move the RF and LF away from each other

Arch B, raising PV and pressing knees towards floor

CRAWLING

Improving walking

Standing on feet and hands, arms and legs straight-ish

Flex and extend the spine, head to tail

Homolateral/contralateral walk

Take straight RL through gap between LF and LH

Take straight LL through gap between RF and RH

On hands and knees

Take bent RL through the gap between LK and LH

Take bent LL through the gap between RK and RH

Cross bent RL over LK

Cross bent LL over RK

Cross bent RL over LK and sit back on heels

Cross bent LL over RK and sit back on heels

Cross bent RL over LK and sit back between feet

Cross bent LL over RK and sit back between feet

Cross bent RL over LK, sit back between feet, and roll onto back

Cross bent LL over RK, sit back between feet, and roll onto back

Cross bent RL over LK, sit back between feet, and roll onto back, then roll back up into sitting between heels

Cross bent LL over RK, sit back between feet, and roll onto back, then roll back up into sitting between heels

Cross bent RL over LK, then take LL from behind RL and bring it round and cross it over RK, then take RL from behind LL and bring it round and cross it over LK, and so on

BUTT-WALKING

Improving walking

Sitting with only left buttock on firm chair with knees and hips at right angles, hands on knees

Raise and lower RBK (and so, RHJ up and down), that is, SBL and SBR

SBL looking up to the left and SBR looking down to the right

Reach over H with RH to left ear, SBL and SBR

Reach over H with LH to right ear, SBL and SBR

Move RK (and so, RHJ) forward and back

Move RHJ in clockwise circles

Move RHJ in counter-clockwise circles

Repeat above sequence **sitting with only right buttock on chair**

Sitting on chair with knees and hips at right angles

Tap RBK/LBK on chair by SBR

Move RHJ/LHJ forward and back

Move LHJ forward and back

Move RHJ in clockwise circles

Move LHJ in clockwise circles

Move RHJ in counter-clockwise circles

Move LHJ in counter-clockwise circles

Move RHJ in clockwise circle, then LHJ in clockwise circle

Move RHJ in counter-clockwise circle, then LHJ in counter-clockwise circle

Butt-walk forward and back

SITTING CROSS-LEGGED

Sitting with LL long, RL frog-legged, RF near BK, hands holding RF, move the RF in circles with hands

Repeat above sequence with LF, the **body arranged oppositely**

Semi-supine

Outside of left ankle on RK, LK pointing out, flex and extend the spine, exhaling with flexion, inhaling with extension

Outside of left ankle on RK, LK pointing out, bring the legs over the RC holding RK with hands, flex and extend spine

Repeat two sequences with the **body arranged oppositely**

Supine

Frog-legged, both feet near BK, hold RF with RH, LF with LH, flex and extend spine

Frog-legged, both feet near BK, hold RF with RH, LF with LH, arch back, raising PV and pressing knees towards floor

Sitting frog-legged

Lift RF towards face and move RF in circles with hands

Lift LF towards face and move LF in circles with hands

Bring mouth towards RK and along RL to RF and over to the LF and along LL to the LK

Sit cross-legged both ways

SERPENTINE SPINE

(Find four 8" x 11" children's picture books)

Semi-supine, LL extended towards ceiling, book on sole of LF

Flex and extend LL

Roll the trunk left and right

Repeat above sequences with book on RF

Semi-supine, LL extended towards ceiling, book on sole of LF, LA extended to ceiling, book on flat LH

Roll the trunk left and right

Repeat above sequence with books on RF and RH

Prone, LK bent at 90°, book on LF

Roll trunk left and right, raise and lower leg, tilt leg right and left, and make circles with LF

Repeat above sequence with book on RF

Semi-supine, LL extended towards ceiling, book on sole of LF, LA extended towards ceiling, book on flat LH

Roll onto front and then back onto back

Repeat above sequence with books on RF and RH

Semi-supine, both legs extended towards ceiling, books on soles of feet, both arms extended towards ceiling, books on flat hands

Roll onto front and then onto B and back onto front and so on – while breathing!

REACHING WITH THE RIBCAGE

Improving the use of the arms

Semi-supine

Straight arms extended above the shoulders, tap right shoulder blade on floor → AND then left shoulder blade → then each alternately

Side-lying on left side

Arms straight in front of shoulders, palms together, slide RA forward, then back → then back and forth

RA lying along right side, move tip of RS forward → then back → then back and forth → then up → then down → then up and down → then in clockwise circles → then in counter-clockwise circles

Slide RK and RHJ forward → then back → then back and forth → then up → then down → then up and down → then in clockwise circles → then in counter-clockwise circles

Slide RHJ forward, RS back → then RHJ back, RS forward

Reach over H with RA to touch left ear and side-bend right

Move RHJ and RS in clockwise circles → then counter-clockwise circles

Extend RA above H, RL below PV and reach up with RA and down with RL, lengthening right side → then shorten right side by hiking up RHJ and drawing RS down, bringing RHJ and RS towards each other

Reach with arms behind and take hold of ankles and make yourself into a bow by working towards straightening legs

Repeat above sequences **side-lying right**

BRIDGING

Semi-supine, extend LL, place RH flat on the floor next to right ear with RE flexed and pointing to the ceiling, wrist extended, and fingers pointing down (towards the feet)

Push with the RF such that the PV rolls left and B extends → slide H through the gap between RS and RH

Repeat sequence with the **body arranged oppositely**

Semi-supine, hands by their respective ears as above

Push with the RF, rolling PV left, extending back, and take the H through the gap between the RS and RH, and then do the opposite, pushing with the LF, extending the B, rolling the PV right, and taking the H through the gap between the LS and LH

Semi-supine, place both hands by their respective ears

Push with both feet, raising PV and arching B

Push with both feet, raising PV and arching B, pause, and then walk the shoulders towards the feet

Push with both feet, raising PV and arching B, pause, and then walk the shoulders and feet until the elbows come alternately to the floor

Push with both feet, raising PV and arching B, and walk the shoulders and feet until elbows come to the floor, take a big breath, hold it, and push the ball of air into the belly and pull it up into the chest

Semi-supine

Push with both feet, raising PV and arching B, and walk the shoulders towards the feet to take hold of the ankles

FORWARD ROLL

Kneeling, fingers interlaced behind H, crown of H on floor

Round the back so that the back of H and neck come to floor

Round the back so that the H and neck come to the floor, pause, and slide the RA through the gap between the LK and LE and RS comes to the floor → then extend LL, rounding back

Repeat above sequence with LA through gap and RL extending

Semi-supine

Bring bent RL over RC and drop the foot to the floor

Bring bent LL over RC and drop the foot to the floor

Bring both bent legs over RC and drop the feet to the floor

Sitting, feet standing, arms wrapped behind knees

Roll onto B and drop feet

Roll onto B and back to sitting

Roll onto B and further onto shoulders and back to sitting

Kneeling, hands in push-ups position, crown of H, on floor

Round the back so that the H and neck come to the floor, then extend legs, rounding back → walk feet forward → and roll and drop the feet to the floor → and reverse the roll

SITTING TO STANDING

Sitting on firm chair with knees and hips at right angles

Tilt forward and back on sitting bones, back firm → a piece of paper could be removed from under BK

Interlace fingers on H and move the scalp back and forth, side to side, in clockwise and counter-clockwise circles until the spine follows

Place back of RH on forehead, palm of LH behind H, and turn H side to side → reverse hands and continue

Sitting, fingers interlaced on H with the fingers inside the palms, relax the arms such that the arms fix the hands on H

Flex and extend the spine, H to tail

Rotate the spine, turning the trunk left and right

Sitting, RH on floor between feet, LH pointing to ceiling

Move the LH in circles such that the extended arms make a cone shape in space → reverse the circles

Repeat the above sequence with the **body arranged oppositely**

Sitting, arms extended above H, fingers interlaced

Tilt forward to comfortable limit and twist the body side to side

Sitting, thumbs under the chin, fingers under occiput

Flex and extend spine/side-bend right and left/butt-walk/tilt forward and back – without putting any weight on the hands

Come to standing without putting any weight on the hands

HATHA YOGA
A Somatic Approach

Awareness, when prioritized, is the essence of what makes yoga *somatic* and fundamentally different from what might be called a *formal* approach. The formal approach attempts to duplicate the form of the pose as conceived from the outside and is purposed, in a sense, to impose or force the *asana* on the body rather than self-organizing the pose as the body. Forcing undermines the integrity of mind and body, which the somatic approach assumes and exemplifies.

A *somatic* approach thus qualifies the *formal* approach:

- engaging every pose in an attitude of exploration

- understanding, organizing and feeling any pose as a whole-body coordination

- defining the pose by its functional and structural purposes rather than by its form, the form a guide to its purposes

- understanding every pose as an approximation of or approach to the form of the pose, staying within a range that is easy

- accomplishing this approximation by feeling into the form

- using the easy limits reached in the approximation to any pose as a means to refine awareness of one's patterns

- returning attention to the sensory effects of this approximation and using those effects to inform the work of feeling towards the form

- and this by pressing or contracting, releasing or undoing, rather than forcing or stretching

- approaching every pose in light of the Weber–Fechner principle whereby the pose is framed as 'speaking loudly' to the limitation or to the challenge that the pose addresses

- approaching each asana with sensitivity - that is, using feedback in terms of discomfort as a guide to practice

- conceiving the pose as a kind of 'intentional stress', a 'confining' manipulation that asks for a somatic adaptation

- using the form of the pose as seen from the outside as a guide to feel on the inside for what is to be toned by pressing or contracting and what is to be toned by lengthening.

STRETCHING

It is impossible to stretch a muscle. The electrochemical bonds that make for muscle contraction have the binding force of tensile steel and are too powerful for any self-applied mechanical force to pull apart. When one 'stretches' muscle, one is in fact stimulating the Golgi tendon receptors by putting the associated tendons on stretch. The brain may interpret this information as increased contraction of the associated muscles, which may thereby reflexively release to their 'normal' measure of tone.

According to Thomas Hanna, a muscle that is not being used for movement, support or in response to gravity ideally has zero tone. By tendency however, a person may have a 'normal' level of muscular tonus that can be as much as 60–80 percent of the measure of contractibility of the muscle. Chronically co-contracted muscle tonus in the elderly is sometimes one of the causes of their apparent weakness.

When tension is put on the tendons in a stretch the brain may perceive thereby that the associated muscle is contracting beyond its established 'normal' and may reduce the stimulus to the muscle in order to release the apparent level of contraction to that familiar 'normal'. (Too great a stretch on the tissue may tear the muscle belly or tear the associated ligaments or tendon or stimulate the stretch reflex, a neurological mechanism that protects muscles from damage: any time that you stretch muscle fibres too far or too suddenly beyond their usual length, this spinal cord reflex contracts those very muscles to protect their integrity. Thus, over-stretching tightens the very muscles you are seeking to release.) Stretching then does not change function so that when one re-engages ordinary action the subcortical habit will tend to reassert itself and the 'normal' level of muscular tonus return.

A limitation in stretching any 'tight muscle' is that such an approach is piecemeal. Unless the release of the musculature is contextualized with respect to a functional pattern, the likelihood of its lasting is minimal for, as Feldenkrais opined, an unresolved part of a problematic pattern tends to reinstitute the whole pattern. If one produces a lowering of muscle tonus through a yoga practice, to establish the new lowered tonus as a functional option it should be reinforced through association with competent movement.

When stretching, you want to go to the point where you feel a mild tension and then relax as you hold the stretch. The feeling of tension should subside quickly as you hold the position. If it does not, you should ease off to a degree of tension that is comfortable and within which you can in fact relax.

Although it is not possible to stretch a muscle you can stretch connective tissue, which becomes stiff with dehydration or lack of use. This even happens overnight to some extent. It certainly happens with a sedentary lifestyle. Part of yoga's purpose is to keep the connective tissue mobile. Stretching of the connective tissue may also serve alignment and symmetry.

The effectiveness of such a discipline as Hatha yoga lies in its comprehensive address to bodily organization, the variety of poses, and its repetition and development with practice. In addition, many yoga poses require the strong tonic contraction of certain muscles. Conscious contraction of muscles is an effective means for learning how to release them.

Although use and functioning are not directly addressed in Hatha yoga, the structure is released and reorganized in such practice. Natural function may thus be more readily attained.

B.K.S. Iyengar wrote in *Light on Yoga* that the goal of Hatha yoga practice is to make the body limber, strong and aligned. The argument in favour of a *somatic* rather than a *formal* approach to that end is that the somatic approach works more gently and effectively by its indirectness and by its engagement of the individual as a self-aware and self-governing agent. A somatic approach will tend to allow for greater functional control and freedom and to increase sensitivity where a formal approach may decrease sensitivity.

ALIGNMENT AND SYMMETRY

Misalignment that involves the myofascia or the skeleton requires compensatory functional adaptations for the mechanism to carry out any action, which will establish habitual patterns in the use of the muscles. Yoga works towards structural realignment via refashioning the connective tissue. Thus, it is important that one balances the work in one-sided poses and antagonistic poses.

When misalignment is of a mild structural nature or caused by a malcoordination due to a functional pattern, it can often be resolved effectively through sensorimotor work. Even in such cases, yoga is helpful.

Realignment was one of the effects of Alexander's early work on himself and produced unfamiliar feelings. These and the consequent tendency to return to what is familiar are obstacles to changing patterns of use. Habits will tend to reassert themselves mechanically as cows will tend to wander down the same path to their watering hole even if the fences are removed and the pasture is wide.

The brain seeks symmetry in feeling and movement. In functional work, symmetry comes about indirectly as a gradual effect of the work. In yoga, one can make that direction conscious by feeling towards symmetry.

An obstacle to structural realignment is the influence of so-called extensile ligaments, which are really small skeletal muscles held at relatively static lengths by motor neurons firing a continuous train of nerve impulses. Most such ligaments are postural muscles in the torso. They have greater elasticity than connective tissue ligaments because of their muscular nature but they function to maintain posture like ordinary ligaments. However, they do not always allow the joints their full range of motion.

Unlike connective tissue ligaments, extensile ligaments are embedded with motor neurons and respond to nerve impulses. Since every muscle associated with the vertebral column is represented on both sides of the body, the matching muscles in each pair should receive the same number of nerve impulses per second in any bilaterally symmetrical posture. If that number is unequal, the paired muscles will develop chronically unequal lengths, which will cause repercussions through the central axis of the body. This condition is a source of right–left musculoskeletal imbalances. Axial imbalances may be evident throughout the torso and vertebral column but are especially noticeable in the neck where the tiny suboccipital muscles function as extensile ligaments to maintain head position. If the head is chronically twisted or tipped to one side it may be that the paired muscles on the two sides have been held at unequal lengths over a long period of time, motor neurons have become habituated to long-established firing patterns, the bellies of the muscles themselves have become shorter on one side and longer on the other, and connective tissue fibres within and surrounding the muscle have adjusted to the unequal lengths of the muscle fibres. In cases of this kind a course of chiropractic adjustments in conjunction with somatic and structural work may be an option.

As Feldenkrais quipped, the closer one gets to the core of the body, the closer one gets to the idiot within. Many yoga poses challenge this issue directly in their demand for conscious and complex muscle contraction and de-contraction through the core: the muscles of the back, the spine, neck and pelvis, the hips and the shoulder girdle.

Many *asanas* demand muscles to be used strongly. If used as a somatic strategy it works on the same principles as strong tonic contraction and pandiculation by providing great sensory input to the associated muscles such that, in so using them, freeing them becomes more available. Such *asanas* provide strong sensory input from the motor effort required to assume and hold the pose. When attention is recalled from the goal of assuming the pose to the somatic event greater benefit accrues. This makes the work a conscious learning process.

Because a pose is felt and moved into slowly and sustained for a period of time, awareness is more easily applied than in the process of complex rapid movements.

PAIN AS INFORMATION

Not all pain is bad. Pain is bad if the system reflexively reacts to it or if it is a sign of damaged tissues. If there is any sense in your judgment that a pain is damaging or if you cannot relax in it you should avoid the movement or position that causes it.

Sometimes the pain and its cause may have been there for some time and it is now, as you are becoming more sensitive to yourself through somatic work, that it comes to your attention. It may be an old pain that is resurfacing as a result of the unwinding of more superficial patterns that have covered it. Sometimes pains are growing pains: as a result of the reorganization of movement, muscles begin to work differently or connective tissue readapts to the changes in organization and causes temporary discomforts. Sometimes it is a chronic pain that is easily triggered because the neural pathway is triggered to fire at the least stimulation. Sometimes it is pain that has been avoided by avoiding positions or movements that stimulate it. Finally, some pain is unavoidable because it is caused by inflammation of the associated tissue.

In all these cases, Alexander's admonition was to 'talk to it nicely'. Find it out through sensitive exploration. A right approach will generally yield a right result and the consequent resolution of symptoms in time.

While yoga offers many of the benefits of high-impact aerobics and body-building in that it stimulates the cardiovascular and respiratory systems, it poses none of the risks if approached intelligently. Yoga should not distress the joints or the connective tissues but rather test them to their benefit.

The regimen presented here works to free the whole body. The forward-bending poses should balance the backward-bending poses, the lateral bends and the twists equally. Each individual will find in time new poses to add to address his or her unique patterning. Once you have grasped the means of working somatically, from the inside out, seeking to refine self-sensing and self-organization, such further exploration of the practice is made easier and more effective.

Some of the illustrations suggest a first approach to the full pose. Similarly, you want to think out a first approach to each pose using the form and purposes as guides.

GENERAL INSTRUCTIONS

The senior principle of somatic yoga is your thoughtful approach to each pose, understanding its theme and purpose. Frame the pose as a shaping of the whole body, conceived as a matrix of the five cardinal lines. Feel and think towards its form. A pose is defined by its purpose, guided by its form. We are not trying to exactly duplicate the form of the pose but rather exploring its purpose through approaching the form. Bring your attention to the areas contracted, toned and released: these are the foreground in the practice and stimulate exploration.

Enough time must be taken in any pose, usually a minute or two, to scan the body thoroughly, becoming attentive to the mass of sensory information stimulated by the pose, considering and sensing, via that information, the address one is making to the purposes of the pose and thereby adjusting oneself accordingly. One is thus only approximating the form, feeling towards one's limit. That limit can be identified by feeling the muscle and connective tissue that is 'on stretch' having a good measure of tone.

In working towards one's limit in a stretching pose or the stretching aspect of a pose one is to relax at one's present-time limit. If one cannot relax into the pose, one has stretched too far. In working towards one's limit in a pressing pose or the pressing aspect of a pose, one is to engage more of oneself in the organization of the pose.

When moving into or out of the pose and when in the pose, check that the breathing is undisturbed. Even strenuous poses are to be guided by this principle.

The freedom of the head–neck relationship and the integrity of the spine are paramount. The question may arise how one can, in a back-bending pose, both follow the direction given in the Alexander Technique to release the head forward and up from the neck and, in the approximation to the pose, let the head hang back and down. The freedom of the head's relationship with the neck is primary to its position. In a backbend then, the head may hang freely such that a release of the axial line and the consequent possibility of a whole-body release are potentiated.

Complete your practice with a lengthy period of *savasana* or dead pose. Like the rests in ATM, *savasana* provides a time for the nervous system to integrate the changes wrought by the practice. *Savasana* may be used after each pose. Semi-supine, even with the bent lower legs supported passively, is also a viable alternative to *savasana*.

ARC

Prone, hands interlaced behind the head. Raise the head, arms, trunk and legs, straight at knees and touching throughout their length.

Purposes and instructions

This pose strongly engages the extensor musculature from the head to the backs of the arms and hands to the soles of the feet; lengthens the spine in extension; and opens and releases the frontal line, especially the belly, solar plexus and throat.

Interlace the fingers behind the head. Look for a congruent tone throughout the front and back. Go up slowly, hold and come down slowly. Breathe evenly especially into the abdomino-thoracic area at the level of the intercostal arch and into the ribcage under the armpits. Repeat several times. Work to increase the degree of the arch of the back and the raising of the elbows, working to bring everything but the pubic bone and belly from the floor.

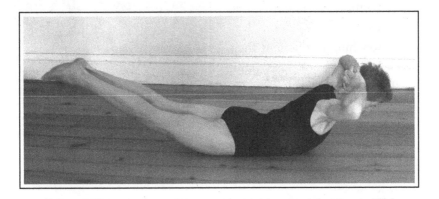

(The limitation of a picture as a communication of what the practice is in the context of yoga or any somatic work is that a picture cannot illustrate the dynamic nature of the pose or movement or the workings of the mind applied to the sensorimotor processes or the subject's idiosyncratic structure.)

PLOUGH

1. Supine, arms by the sides, the shoulders supported on a folded blanket to ease the stretch on the neck. Swing the legs overhead onto a chair seat. Straighten the legs.

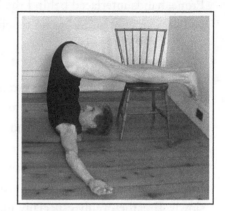

2. Supine, arms extended at shoulder height. Swing the legs overhead, bringing the knees to the floor by the ears.

3. Supine. Swing the legs overhead, straightening them, bringing the feet to the floor, legs touching throughout their length. Lock the chin into the jugular notch. Interlace the fingers and extend the straight arms behind the back. Extend the legs via the heels.

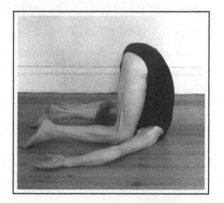

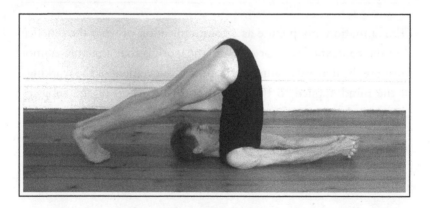

Purposes and instructions

This pose lengthens and relaxes the back in flexion from the head to the feet, especially the neck and upper back, low back and buttocks. Allow and feel for a congruent lengthening and tone throughout the back from the head through the soles of the feet to the toes. Bring the whole back into your awareness. Relax the neck, shoulders and back. Relax the belly, the front of the neck and tongue. Let the breath move into the back.

CROSS

Supine. Arms spread wide at shoulder height, raise the legs and straighten them perpendicular to the ceiling. Tilt the legs very slowly to the side and hold. Increase the angle of the legs until the feet nearly touch the floor.

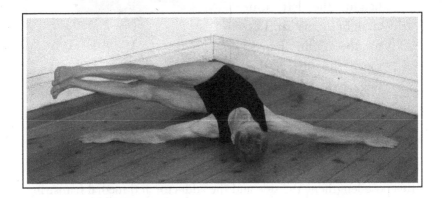

Purposes and instructions

This pose lengthens and strengthens the abdominal oblique muscles and lengthens the spine in lateral rotation. Work to keep the neck and back long, the lower back flat, the buttocks relaxed, the opposite shoulder down – the lateral rotation happening mainly at the hip joints, sacroiliac joints and lumbar spine. Breathe evenly. Keep the frontal line open. Use the slow eccentric contraction of the muscles of the waist and back to allow their releasing and toning.

TRIANGLE

1. Standing, feet spread wide, the right foot turned out at 90 degrees, the right arm extended at shoulder height, the left arm straight by the ear. Tilt to the right.

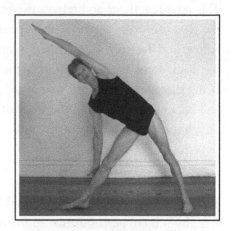

2. Standing, feet spread wide, the right foot turned out at 90 degrees, the right arm extended at shoulder height, the left arm straight by the ear. Tilt to the right. Barely touch the tips of the fingers to the floor. Do not bear weight through the hand.

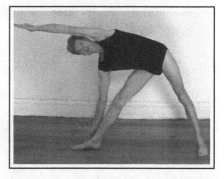

Purposes and instructions

This pose lengthens the side and the adductor and medial hamstring muscles of the leg, opens the hips in abduction and lateral rotation, strengthens the muscles of the trunk and laterally lengthens the spine. Keep the pelvis and face facing forward and the spine straight, the chest released up, the shoulders relaxed. Spread the toes and keep the fingers together. Draw the kneecaps up and keep the knees unlocked. Allow the eccentric contraction of the muscles of the side and leg to release and tone them. Keep the belly relaxed and moving with the breath. Repeat on both sides.

REVERSE TRIANGLE

Standing, the feet spread wide, the right foot turned out at 90 degrees, the left in to 45 degrees, the arms extended at shoulder height. Rotate the trunk 180 degrees. Tilt to the left. Barely touch the tips of the fingers to the floor. Do not bear weight through the hand.

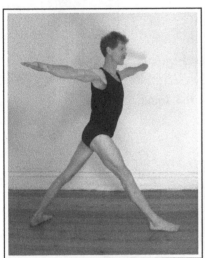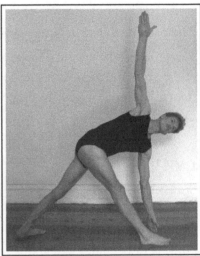

Purposes and instructions

This pose lengthens the oblique muscles of the waist, lengthens the spine in rotation, mobilizes the hips, tests balance and strengthens the muscles of the trunk. Spread the toes and keep the fingers together, the shoulders relaxed, the spine 'straight', the frontal line open, the arms released out of the ribcage via the shoulder girdle and supported by the trunk. Keep the face in the same direction as the chest. Draw the kneecaps up and keep the knees unlocked. Seek lengthening and tone in the waist, back and buttocks. Repeat both ways.

EAGLE

Standing on the left foot, wind the arms, left over right, the palms together, and wind the legs, right over left, the right foot hooked around the left ankle, squat and balance. Face forward.

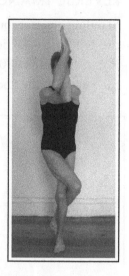

Purposes and instructions

This pose tests balance and mobilizes the joints of the arms and legs. Keep the body erect, the frontal line open. Work to deepen the squat. Do both ways.

TWIST

Seated, the left leg sharply bent, the right knee bent, foot standing left of the left knee, right hand behind. Twist the trunk, taking hold of the right big toe with the left hand.

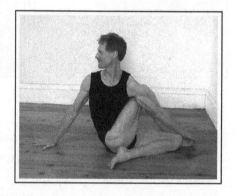

Purposes and instructions

This pose lengthens the spine in rotation and mobilizes the hips and shoulders. Balance the weight equally on both sitting bones and keep the line between them at right angles to the direction of the thighs. Keep the chest up and open, the spine erect. Release the neck. Think of using the arms and shoulders as the levers by which to twist the axial line from the hips to the head. Do the twist in both directions.

COBBLER

Seated, leaning easily on the hands behind, bring the soles of the feet together and draw the knees down towards the floor. Keep the back straight and as vertical as possible. Use high firm cushions or low bench under the buttocks to start.

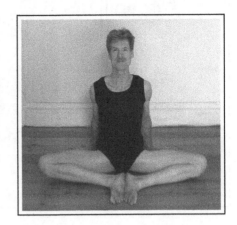

Purposes and instructions

This pose opens the hips in abduction and stretches the ligaments of the knees. Press the knees down while keeping the pelvis rotated forward onto the sitting bones, the chest up. Breathe evenly into the belly.

COW

1. Seated on a chair, the spine erect, the left foot on the opposite thigh, reach overhead with the right hand holding a belt, the left hand behind the back to catch the belt.

2. Seated on the right foot, spine erect, the legs wound around each other, lift the left hand behind the back to catch the belt.

3. Seated on floor between the feet, weight balanced between the buttocks, spine erect, the legs wound around each other, left over right, reach overhead with the right hand, the left hand behind back, hold the hands.

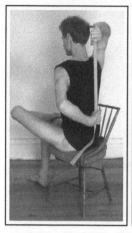 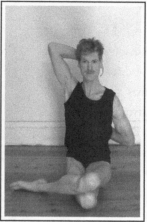 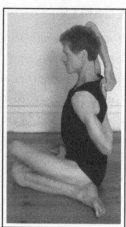

Purposes and instructions

This pose opens the hips in adduction, and the chest and shoulders in extension. Keep the neck free and aligned with the spine, the chest open and up, the shoulder girdle released from the ribcage, the back broad. Let the weight sink through into the sitting bones, releasing the hip joints. Bear weight evenly on both buttocks. Reverse the legs and arms.

GORILLA

Standing, the feet spread wide, flexed at hips, hands between feet, arms and legs straight, back arched, face forward.

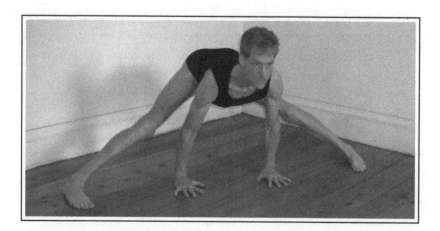

Purposes and instructions

This pose opens the hips in abduction, tones the adductors, opens the frontal line and opens the shoulders in retraction. Ensure the pelvis is even. Release the hips backwards. Keep the kneecaps drawn up and the knees unlocked. Spread the toes and fingers and bear weight through the hands and feet. Work to increase the width of the stance.

HANDSTAND

Standing facing the wall, bend forward placing the hands about shoulder width apart, 5 to 10 inches from the wall, swing the feet overhead, straightening the legs.

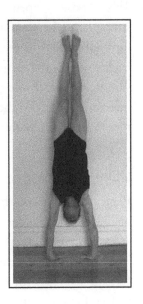

Purposes and instructions

This pose opens and strengthens the arms and shoulders, tests balance and extends the wrists. Work to keep the neck free and the breathing regular. Ensure that the balls of the fingers are pressing into the floor. Extend the arms out of the chest via the shoulder girdle. Work to keep the trunk firm and straight.

DOWNWARD DOG

1. Plant the feet shoulder width apart at a distance from a chair or table top such that hinging only at the hips allows the hands to press upon the chair.

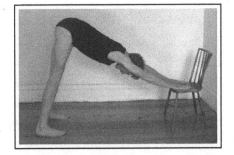

2. Plant the feet shoulder width apart and, hinging only at the hips, plant the hands on the floor about shoulder width apart.

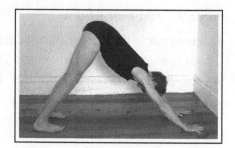

Purposes and instructions

This pose opens and strengthens the shoulders, extends the back and front, and frees the hips and ankles in flexion. Work to keep the neck released and the back straight, the arms in line with the back. Breathe evenly. Make sure that the full sole of the foot and palm of the hand are pressing into the floor. Keep the frontal line open. Seek length and tone from toes to head. Draw the kneecaps up and keep the knees unlocked.

LION

Plant the hands and the balls of the feet shoulder width apart in push-ups position, supporting weight with arms. Extend the back powerfully to face forwards, turning the feet onto their tops.

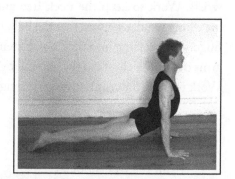

Purposes and instructions

This pose strengthens the shoulders, opens the chest, stretches the spine in extension and frees the ankles and wrists. Keep the neck free, the throat and chest open, the gaze upwards and the trunk and legs firm. Draw the shoulders back and lift the trunk out of the shoulders. Breathe evenly. Work for length and tone from toes through the whole front to the head.

FORWARD BEND

1. Seated, the legs straight over a rolled towel, hinge forward only at the hips and grasp the big toes with the index fingers.

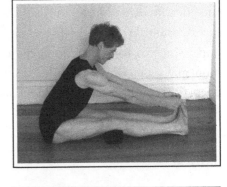

2. Seated, the legs straight over a rolled towel, hinge forward only at the hips and interlace the fingers under the soles of the feet.

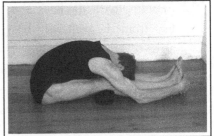

Purposes and instructions

This pose lengthens the spine in flexion, opens the hip joints in flexion, lengthens the back from the head, neck, back, buttocks and legs to the feet, and mobilizes the shoulders. Release the hips. Keep the spine integrated so that the bending is taken in the hips. Breathe evenly into the back. The rolled towel prevents hyperextension of the knee. Seek a relaxed toning of the whole back of the body.

CAMEL

Kneel with the tops of the feet on the floor, the hands on the soles of the feet, the heels of the hands on the heels of the feet, extend the back and neck powerfully, extending the pelvis forward.

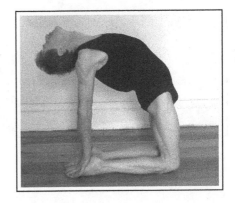

Purposes and instructions

This pose stretches the knees and ankles, opens the frontal line and shoulders in extension, and relaxes the neck and lengthens the spine in extension. Work to keep the neck free, allowing the head and upper spine to hang back from the chest. Draw the shoulders back more and more. Breathe evenly into the solar plexus. Keep the throat open, the mouth closed, the face relaxed. Look for a lengthening tone from the knees to the head.

BRIDGE

1. Standing with the back about two feet from the wall, lean back with arms overhead and bear weight with the hands on the wall, fingers pointing down. Walk down the wall with the hands only as far as you can and still bring yourself back up.

2. Supine, knees bent, feet standing, the legs touching throughout their length, hands by the ears, fingers pointing down, raise the body into an arch. Bring the elbows to the floor, fingers interlaced cupping the head. Press the floor with the elbows.

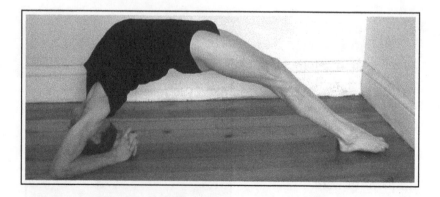

Purposes and instructions

This pose opens the frontal line and the shoulders, strengthens the muscles of the trunk and lengthens the spine in extension. Breathe evenly into the solar plexus. Keep the neck free and the face relaxed. Push strongly through the shoulders into the arms or elbows, minimizing the weight through the head. Work to bring the extension high up into the upper chest and spine. Look for a lengthening tone from the front of the ankles to the elbows.

HEAD–KNEE BEND

1. Seated, the right leg straight over a rolled towel, the left foot on the right thigh, spine straight, loop a belt around the right foot, hinge forward from the sitting bones.

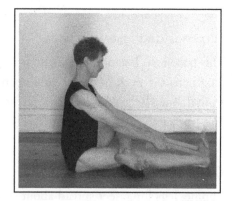

2. Seated, the right leg straight over a rolled towel, the left foot on the right thigh, spine straight, bend forward from the sitting bones, taking hold of the right foot with the hands, the forehead on the knee.

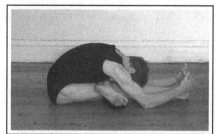

Purposes and instructions

This pose lengthens the back in flexion, opens the hips in outward rotation and flexion, and opens the shoulders in extension. Keep the spine long, the frontal line open from the sitting bones to the throat. Work to differentiate the legs from the pelvis at the hip joints. Seek length and tone from the toes to the head. Let the buttocks open. Release the whole back of the body from the back of the neck through the legs to the soles of the feet and toes. Switch the legs. The rolled towel prevents hyperextension of the knee.

CANDLE

Supine, swing the legs overhead into the Plough pose. Support the upper back with the hands. Bring the whole body to perpendicular. Tuck the chin into the jugular notch.

Purposes and instructions

This pose tests balance, opens the shoulders, lengthens the neck in flexion and opens the frontal line. Relax the neck, buttocks, legs and trunk.

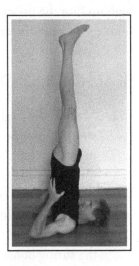

CORPSE

Supine, legs long, feet spread about shoulder width apart, arms long, shoulder blades flat on floor, palms up.

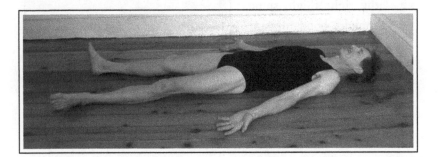

Purposes and instructions

This pose serves to integrate the changes from the practice. Consciously release the body, from top to bottom and bottom to top, and repeat the process until you are maximally relaxed. Relax the breath. Relax thinking. Relax attention. Rest completely and be simply awake before things happen.

Questions and Answers

ISN'T GOOD POSTURE REALLY JUST A MATTER OF HOLDING ONESELF PROPERLY?

A common misconception about posture is that it exists. A second misconception about posture is that it matters. A third is that you can do something directly about it.

First, no posture that one assumes, even 'standing still', is altogether static. That is why 'acture', connoting the always-dynamic response to gravity, is a preferable term.

Second, 'correcting' a static pose cannot significantly affect what a person does when they are active. In fact, it is not useful to instruct or show someone how to stand 'correctly' and expect that to have any lasting effect on a person's active life because state-specific learning is ineffective. That is, learning is not effective and lasting change if it pertains only under specific circumstances.

Third, the belief that you can correct the way you stand or move and accurately know whether you are in fact correct is downright wrong. If you could correct the way you stand or move by adjusting yourself you would already have done so because you would already be feeling how your movement or coordination is wrong. And you cannot sustain any 'corrections' that you may make because your habitual 'wrong feeling' or faulty self-sensing undermines your deliberate volition to consistently adopt a new form. This was Alexander's critical discovery more than a hundred years ago and the conundrum in which he found himself when he was trying to correct his own use problem. Alexander found, through observing himself and trying to correct his movement by doing something, that it was impossible for him to successfully do so because the very faculty upon which he depended to make his adjustments, his 'self-awareness', was giving him wrong information.

Because the self-senses are interfaced with the movement function in the nervous system self-sensing can go wrong when something goes wrong with movement. So, Alexander discovered that it is not fruitful to correct 'doing' alone but that he had to first re-educate his self-sensing. And this is why not only posture but chronic or recurrent pain, which often results from habitual coordination that is not harmonious with the structure, is such a tricky problem as it too cannot be resolved directly.

If a person knew how to move correctly he would already be doing so. When that is not the case, then he has to learn again to sense what he is doing. It must be emphasized that a person with a pain, posture or use problem is really not presently clearly aware of what he is doing because, if he were, he would already not be doing the thing that is problematic. This paradox is not generally understood or accounted for in conventional treatment of functional problems, whether they are tension or pain, inflexibility or clumsiness, joint disorders, voice or breathing difficulties, spinal problems, post-traumatic or post-surgical limitations and so on. That is why conventional medical treatment is largely ineffective in these areas. The sensorimotor functions do not fall within its field of expertise fundamentally because the sensorimotor process is an holistic process involving the body and the mind-brain-body as totalities whereas the medical paradigm denies the existence or, at least, the importance of the mind and treats the body as a sum of its parts, which it isn't.

Teachers of the Alexander Technique re-educate a person's self-sensing through instruction and with their hands, which hands are uniquely trained to sense subtleties of movement and tension. The teacher's expertise is in his or her ability to best organize, through refined manipulation, the pupil's movement, coordination and response to gravity via an ongoing address to the pupil's core dynamic as which all movement is organized. The teacher guides the person through simple movements while seeking and facilitating the easier way, which facilitation is rooted in the teacher's understanding of and feel for this core dynamic. At the same time, the teacher enlists the individual's innate capability to attend to him- or herself and to become aware of habitual patterning, and stimulates the person's self-exploration and growing capacity for freedom and control of the physical self. The teacher works to ease out chronic action of muscles that are doing too much and coax the appropriate degree of activity from muscles that are under-used. Through thus guided simple activities the pupil learns to free him- or herself from misuse patterns and to allow natural poise and balance to re-emerge. In time, the person becomes able to generalize the practices and principles learned so that lightness and freedom of movement become the common experiences of daily life. 'Acture', the always-dynamic response to gravity, and movement are thus effectively re-educated. Through practice one unlearns faulty habits and relearns right use. A virtuous spiral of improvement is initiated.

WHAT MAKES A MOVEMENT GOOD?

The essence of a good movement is the coordinated use of the whole mechanism to produce an integrated action.

In general, a person tends to bring to the process of any action, in Alexander's words, the same habitual use of himself that he brings to all his actions. Thus, if a person wishes to improve the quality of his movement altogether or of any mechanical skill in particular and it doesn't come naturally it is because his use of himself, how he characteristically moves *and* senses himself, is unreliable and must be re-educated. This re-education must take into account the fact that the way we move, coordinate and use ourselves in general directly produces somatic sensations with respect to how we are moving, which in turn guide our movements.

Each of us moves in a recognizable way. How an individual characteristically organizes his or her movement, whether in daily life or in the performance of any skill, 'feels right'. It must 'feel right'. Otherwise we would move differently. To change the way we organize ourselves requires an uncharacteristic manner of action, which necessarily entails unfamiliar experiences, which experiences will 'feel wrong'.

Alexander says that our desire to feel right in what we do tends to be stronger than our desire to improve the quality of our actions, that although one begins with the desire to move more competently, the opposing habit to repeat sensory experiences of ourselves that feel right acts as a stimulus to use the body in the habitual way that produces those familiar experiences of ourselves, although it is this habitual patterning that prevents our satisfying the newer desire. He says that the habitual way we use ourselves tends to be the dominating influence in our response to our desire to change because this habitual way of using ourselves feels right.

He says that, in order to re-educate the way we use the parts of ourselves in any particular activity, it is necessary to re-educate the way we use ourselves as a whole in every activity, that it is therefore necessary to consider the mechanism as a functional unity in which the working of the parts are a function of the working of the whole.

The first step to learning, Alexander says, is to relinquish the desire to gain the goal of our actions directly because this effort will tend to instigate the habitual use of the mechanisms involved in the process of achieving the goal. By this primary act of relinquishing the desire to gain our end, the way is left clear to attend to the 'means whereby' of our actions and thus to learn a new 'use of the self'.

This understanding is fundamental to human improvement and original to the Alexander Technique.

IS THE ALEXANDER TECHNIQUE A REMEDY FOR ARTHRITIS?

Thomas Hanna once said that he had never in his many years of practice encountered a case of osteoarthritis. Tom said that, instead of 'osteoarthritis', a better word was 'rackafrack'. 'You've got a touch of the rackafrack.' 'What is this pain here, doctor?' 'It's a bit of the rackafrack.' Tom, like F.M. Alexander and Moshe Feldenkrais before him, was prone to hyperbolic speech in order to make a point which most of us need to hear: it is not something you have; it is in your manner of action. In spite of this, such terms as fibromyalgia, regional muscular syndrome, stress, rheumatism and the weather are popular ways of identifying the causes of unidentifiable patterns of human pain.

Even when a person is suffering from real arthritis or musculoskeletal problems, it is only in unusual cases that a person cannot improve his or her condition through sensorimotor learning. The common cause of pain that is not organic in nature is undue muscular contraction. Usually one can trace functional problems to muscular contraction that is superfluous, inappropriate or parasitical to effective movement and responsive acture. This can be remedied because, when things go wrong, we have two great resources to which to turn for renewal: our conscious intelligence and somatic methodology, which has outstripped in the last century the benefits offered by mainstream medical approaches.

It is possible to relearn what we have forgotten in the course of our lives, which is relaxed and flexible efficiency and resilience in the process of everyday action, whereby the way we move is harmonious with our physical structure, thereby bypassing the creation of pain, and conformed to the mechanical requirements of the surrounding world and so, maximally effective.

Alexander, Feldenkrais and Hanna were brilliant educators. The essential nature of their teaching work is similar. Each of their methods is the facilitation of improved self-sensing and movement through sensitive and skilful manipulation and instruction. By improving your ability to feel how you are doing what you are doing, you can unlearn those habits of coordination that involve patterns of undue muscular contraction and relearn a manner of self-organization that removes the stress on the joints and tissues. Then, if there is in fact any organic deterioration the body can begin to heal itself.

In reflex reaction to stressors, movement may become compromised. Because of the inextricable impact of movement on self-sensing, your self-sensing then becomes incomplete. The quality of your movement thus becomes further compromised. Without re-education these dysfunctional habits of self-sensing and moving remain and are the precursors to joint and tissue inflammation and pain. That is why Tom Hanna said that arthritis is not something you have but is in the way you do what you do.

Many people need to re-acknowledge the body's value, reawaken curiosity and become responsible for growth. When we begin to make improvements in function through somatic work we open ourselves to positive transformation. In time, the inherent healing force of Life re-establishes health and the pleasure in bodily being.

WILL THE TECHNIQUE MAKE ME LOOK BETTER?

When you drive through the countryside, you may see a tree's branches swept by the prevailing winds like a woman's hair in a slipstream. The constancy of the wind shapes the tree as it grows through the seasons. The same shaping occurs in our connective tissue by our characteristic patterns of movement and posture.

Even a regular exercise routine does not significantly alter this as it is no match for our chronic patterns of use. Exercise is like an occasional windstorm. In fact, such exercise can exacerbate both the problems of misuse and its consequences, which are practiced harder during exercise.

The Alexander Technique and the Feldenkrais Method offer effective means of learning balanced movement and posture. This is made possible by our having a naturally integrated pattern of biomechanics and a virtually limitless capacity for learning.

The Feldenkrais Method works with the movement-related question: is this or this or that coordination easier for my structure? By exploring differences between related movements and by being called thus to awareness through movement and by finding alternatives to the stressful or ineffective we relearn a more harmonious coordination; flexibility arises from our having more movement options; nothing gets flabby through non-use or over-stressed through imbalance.

The Alexander Technique works with the movement-related question: what am I doing to interfere with the natural pattern? – and answering that question, under the teacher's manual and instructional guidance, by noticing the patterns of interference, un-doing them and allowing the teacher's direction into better self-organization.

From the conventional view there are some six hundred muscles in the body. Thus, in circuit training, there is an address to as many of those muscles as possible. However, the sum of the parts does not make the whole. From the somatic view, the body is one muscle shaped by the structure and one responds always as a totality. This action of the whole body in every moment of action is centrally organized. This central organization of movement is the purview of these two somatic methods.

The Feldenkrais Method facilitates improvement in sensing the whole bodily pattern of movement by taking a function apart and putting it together again. This clarification of movement is founded in the nervous system, which is the central informative organizer of movement. The Alexander Technique frees the primary control of movement, which is the central formative organizer of movement. In clarifying and mastering the primary control functionally integrated action emerges.

Improved appearance is possible through improving the quality of movement. One's characteristic manner of movement, like the West Wind's shaping the pine, shapes the body over time. If one's manner of use comes to be balanced, flexible and integrated with one's structure, that shape becomes functional and naturally attractive.

CAN ELDERLY PEOPLE BENEFIT FROM THESE METHODS?

Consider the consequences of clenching your fist for the next few hours: the hand and arm and eventually even the shoulder, neck, back and chest would begin to hurt. If you were to somehow forget you were contracting the hand, you might come to think that something separate from you is afflicting you, perhaps a disease process of some kind. You would also notice that the options and flexibility available to the open hand are not available to the contracted one. Thus arise the usual signs of ageing – pain, affliction and limitation.

Alexander observed that we tend to develop habits of how and what we feel and of how and what we move. Over time we come to act through patterns of contraction and sensory 'amnesia' rather than with freedom and sensitivity. We overlay mechanically sound responses with misdirected effort. We move ourselves in characteristically limited ways and in patterns of undue tension whose availability to conscious control and feeling has been lost. And we fail to notice that we are responsible for this patterning.

Every time you stand up, you might unknowingly tighten your neck – a not uncommon pattern. After twenty years of doing so, you develop pain in your shoulders, neck or upper back. Your doctor tells you, 'It's a slipped disk,' 'It's arthritis,' 'You're getting old,' 'It's in your family history,' 'It's the rackafrack,' but, in fact, it's in how you do what you do.

We tend not to notice how we use ourselves in movement until we begin to suffer the consequences of this in the forms of pain, stiffness and afflictions that come upon us unexplained, limitations in what we can do or the necessity to curtail our activities. But it is not a problem of ageing but of learning. What we have learned wrongly or traumatically or from faulty adaptation and repetition can be unlearned and better use relearned because there is a natural design of human function evolved over the millions of years of our adaptation to gravity and because each of us has a virtually limitless capacity for learning.

CAN CHIROPRACTIC AND MASSAGE HELP A BAD BACK?

Anyone who has tried chiropractic treatment for a problem neck or back knows that it can provide temporary relief. Chiropractic strives to realign the spine, which realignment does not actually address and resolve the causes of the spine's misalignment. That is, it does not make any changes in muscle tension, habitual patterns of movement or your response to stress.

Acupuncture and shiatsu work to balance meridians or as analgesics and also fail to address the function- and use-related causes of back problems. Physiotherapists and Pilates instructors often train patients to strengthen the abdominal muscles, to 'stabilize the back'. This sets up a vicious spiral of co-contraction whereby the frontal musculature gets stronger, causing the back to work even harder to maintain posture, which in time compresses the body and exacerbates the original back problem. Some physiotherapists advise exercises to tone the back, usually the essence of the problem.

Massage, while helpful, provides only passive partial piecemeal release so that, when one returns to activity, one has no means to practice the relaxation in action because the constant of misuse remains unchanged. Conventional medicine offers drugs, which are only palliative. Eventually the person is given a nerve block, a drug injection or surgery, the latter randomly successful, used only when the problem has caused clinically significant damage. The patient may then feel symptomatic relief whereupon the doctor tells him to now go out and strengthen the back.

The reason for this cycle of pain relief and painful return is that most therapies deal only with symptoms – inflammation, spinal misalignment, nerve impingement, muscle tightness and so forth – not the present causes. The symptoms reappear because these causes have not been addressed. Yet, the present root of our pain and functional problems is often simple: it is in the way we move and sense ourselves.

Whereas it is true that some 80 percent of adults suffer chronic or recurring back pain, 20 percent do not! This is because their use of themselves is naturally better. Still, the rest of us can learn such good use because there is a natural manner of human movement evolved over the millions of years of our adaptation to gravity and because we all have a virtually limitless capacity for learning in the form of the human nervous system, which controls sensing, coordination and movement of the body in general and of the back in particular.

Our backs are not the problem. Rather, we use ourselves badly. As we learn or relearn to use ourselves and our backs better, we cease to compress, distort, overwork, misalign or collapse – and thereby damage – our backs.

The Alexander Technique improves the use of ourselves so that soon not only are we freed of pain but also we have the means to correct ourselves if we are beset by a new functional problem in the course of our lives. We become self-understanding, self-reliant and self-regenerative, knowing our own bodies and capable of our own cure.

WHAT ABOUT PHYSICAL EXERCISE?

Strengthening exercises and aerobics are common methods for attaining functional health. Their fundamental drawback is that they do not address our use.

Your muscle build may conform to some ideal but that ideal rarely provides a useful support to daily activities. You may be fit in terms of cardiopulmonary capacity but be neither breathing well nor relaxed. In spite of such exercise, the manner in which you carry out any common activity tends to remain founded on your habitual self-organization, which may be ineffective and harmful.

Conventional exercise seldom facilitates functionally useful improvement. In fact, it can aggravate inefficient patterns and lead to stiffness, pain, fatigue and the rackafrack. Efficient action in contrast is inherently pleasurable, aesthetically pleasing and regenerative.

If you are somatically self-aware then you have effective control of the musculature. It can be used optimally in response to an intention to act and otherwise be relaxed. Relaxed musculature is the essence of flexibility. You are also more sensitive to yourself so that when tension arises or you find yourself going wrong, you can then feel how to undo your pattern of tension or find a better response.

When you learn to use all of yourself in an harmonious way you bring into action the unified strength of the whole body. So, in lifting, for example, all of the body's musculature will participate harmoniously, not just the arms and back. Six hundred-odd muscles working thus together as one are stronger than several dozen. Moreover, optimally released musculature is effectively stronger than chronically over-toned musculature because a released muscle has more available contractibility. When the anti-gravity mechanisms are working reflexively, the body buoyant and relaxed, and ease rather than effort the context of every action, the heart works without strain and the body is allowed full breathing.

Somatic learning methods are more interesting, more pleasurable and more life-affirming than body-building and circuit training where you are effectively fighting your own body. Effortlessness is both the means and the goal of somatic methods. They are uniquely modern and scientifically sound.

MY PHYSIOTHERAPIST TELLS ME TO STRENGTHEN MY ABDOMINAL MUSCLES TO STABILIZE MY BACK: IS THAT CORRECT?

From dance teachers to Pilates instructors, body-builders to physiotherapists comes the admonition to tighten the abdominal muscles. Tight or highly toned abdominal muscles in fact work against the functional health of the body. The abdominal musculature consists of the rectus abdominus muscle that, when over-toned, produces the washboard effect and that runs from the pubic bone to the middle ribs and the internal and external oblique and the transversus muscles that wrap around and give shape to the waist. The main functions of these muscles are to contain the viscera and assist in balance. They do that reflexively and are rightly toned in that process if the person is otherwise well organized in his or her dynamic response to gravity. Their secondary functions are assisting in the twisting and turning of the body during movement and initiating forward flexion of the trunk.

Exercising, as repetitive movement against resistance in the form of an apparatus (weights) or of gravity (sit-ups and such) or of one's own antagonistic musculature (isometrics) is of little benefit to the tonic support mechanisms.

Strengthening the frontal musculature and habituating its shortening requires more work from the musculature of the back in order to maintain upright balance. This causes a vertical compression of the body and thickening of the waist through the resultant shortening of the back and the front and contributes to back pain by overworking the back and compressing the intervertebral disks.

Increasing tone paradoxically reduces strength. Muscles are strongest at their full natural length. Thus, a body that is always optimally released is functionally stronger and, of course, more comfortable.

Tight abdominal muscles are analogous to the corsets that women wore in the past. They cause deterioration of the back, they restrict breathing, they interfere with the working of the viscera, and they bow to fashion to the detriment of health.

Ideally, with each inspiration, the diaphragm is drawn down, the lower ribs expand outwards, and the viscera are pushed down and out, all this as the abdominal muscles reflexively relax. With 'tight abs', the diaphragm cannot descend fully and the lower ribcage cannot expand, so breathing is restricted. The long-term effects of diminished respiration can be chronic fatigue, depression, asthma and any number of other consequences of inadequate oxygenation of the blood. Tight abs compress the viscera, which can interfere with digestion, elimination and the sexual function.

A flat belly is a fad. How can it be right for one's self-esteem to conform to a norm? Remarkably, fear and anxiety are expressed bodily in the contraction of the abdominals. Think of the psychological and cultural consequences of our cultivating and admiring that. Hardening the abdominal musculature may also be associated with armouring oneself against vulnerability or with the compulsion to control one's vital life. And generally it is associated with an effort to look hard, cool and tough, a psychology hardly congruent with cooperation, tolerance and peace.

The viscera are suspended by tough connective tissue, the peritoneal mesentery, from the spine. When the back is lengthening in its response to gravity, the peritoneal mesentery is drawn upwards and backwards with the spine, thereby drawing the viscera up and back.

WILL I ALWAYS HAVE TO WORK ON MYSELF?

In Goddard Binkley's excellent autobiography of lessons with Alexander in his last years (Binkley 1993), Alexander states that if he did not continue to work on himself he would deteriorate.

The body reflects all of its experiences in its patterning and as well the individual's emotional, characteristic, cognitive and egoic strategies, which manifest as patterns of physical self-contraction. The Technique is a means of resolving this patterning.

We are alive as bodies, intelligence and awareness. Obsession about health is probably not appropriate. Yet, finding the right balance *vis-à-vis* functional health in a culture wherein the body has been both eschewed, even demeaned, via the lasting influence of the dominant religious and spiritual perspectives and the usual upbringing, often indulged and exploited through life in reaction to perceived suppression, and otherwise mistreated because of poor education, is a delicate matter that has to be considered intelligently.

We can learn and establish good habits. Through methods such as the Alexander Technique and the Feldenkrais Method, deteriorated functioning is diminished or resolved and improved habits of movement, coordination and acture are realized. We become sensitive. Grace rather than difficulty more and more accompanies our actions. This process of improvement is potentially limitless.

CAN THE TECHNIQUE BE USEFUL IN THE FIELD OF HEALTHCARE?

Alexander's unique discovery and what he determined to be the missing link in medical diagnosis is use. When he demonstrated his method's success in resolving back and neck pain, stutter, poor breathing, asthma, poor posture and other functional disabilities but also so-called idiopathic problems that stumped doctors the Technique was acclaimed by some of the most prestigious members of the British medical profession. But then as now, his work was unable to influence or infiltrate the medical establishment to any significant degree. Any hope of its doing so in our time in the face of the technocracy of modern medicine and the widespread resort to that model and to the methods of symptomatic treatment dominant today is even more remote. And yet, the Alexander Technique offers a uniquely effective alternative and supplement to common healthcare practices.

Use can be defined as the continued exercise of conscious intelligence applied to the organization of function. The limitation of language is how Alexander came upon the use of his hands to give experiences of what he had discovered.

'Manipulation' here indicates the strategies of touch and handling and does not imply brusqueness, force or coercion. In fact, in the Technique, the manipulations are informative rather than formative, and their purposes are freedom, awareness and intelligence in action, purposes radically different from medical modalities.

So what exactly is 'the continued exercise of conscious intelligence applied to the organization of function'?

'Intelligence' is to play, explore, investigate, discriminate, wonder, consider and so on. This is the intelligence to be brought to oneself in the Technique: 'How do I work?'

'Conscious' can be illustrated thus: pay attention to your right big toe. Now, no scientist can test what you just did and that indeed is one of the fundamental limitations of science: it has no access to your and my experience, my awareness of myself, which is obviously real. It is thus also the limitation of medicine, which addresses the body as a 'third-person' event. But it is no limitation on the Technique and its address to the 'first person' event. In fact, that is exactly the purview of the Technique.

The significance of 'application' can be conveyed in this way. For a moment, make a fist. Having made a fist, open the hand. Again, make a fist. Now, do not do that anymore. Remarkably, nobody knows how your intention to make or unmake a fist produces a neuromuscular response. Nobody knows or ever will know how the mind plies the brain.

'Organization' is the dynamic integration of a system.

'Function' refers to our movement, response to gravity, our interaction with the environment and manipulations and our coordination altogether. These combined are use.

Use can be accessed both inwardly, which is the basis for working on oneself, and outwardly, the basis of the hands-on skill of the teacher. This is missing in medical diagnosis. Without it a person must rely on passive treatment, which negates self-responsibility in one's healthcare. Without this responsibility the habits and practices that brought about the degenerative processes associated with ill-health will undermine any passive treatment modalities.

Although a physiotherapist, doctor, massage therapist or chiropractor may move parts of the body as a teacher of the Technique may appear to do the purposes are fundamentally different. An Alexander teacher is seeking to understand how the person is organizing him- or herself in terms of movement and the response to gravity, and to understand how and what the person is thinking and sensing in terms of the mechanics of function. A therapist has no such ideas because such a therapist does not typically conceive of him- or herself as working with sensorimotor intelligence, awareness, freedom and the ability to learn.

The Technique works from the 'outside' as medical science does but, where medicine's approach is symptomatic, the Technique addresses function in a uniquely holistic manner. And unlike medical modalities the Technique works from the 'inside' by facilitating the pupil's own self-exploration, self-awareness and self-understanding and by the teacher's unique ability to use his or her hands to both sense and redirect the dynamics of movement.

Even if you have managed to follow the thesis so far, as Alexander discovered, words remain inadequate to describe a lesson in the Technique. As a picture is worth a thousand words, a lesson, which involves at least six senses, mind and cognition and continuity through time, is impossible to describe. Still, the kind of learning facilitated in an Alexander lesson is natural to us for we have all learned this way in our own development from virtually helpless newborns, capable of only a few simple reflexes, to children who could walk, run, swim, skip, skate and so on, and thence to adults with multiple motor skills.

The Alexander Technique facilitates this kind of sensorimotor learning consciously for many of us have since unconsciously unlearned that natural grace through conditioning factors. Organic diseases have a less easy hold on a fluid body. When a person is free in physical terms, the heart, lungs and viscera have more space and work without restriction. Blood flow is improved. So-called idiopathic hypertension and stress-induced syndromes are obviated in place. Remarkably, these benefits and more have been researched by medical science itself.

The Alexander Technique resolves the functional root of many of the disease processes of modern times. It initiates a regenerative cycle from which spontaneously emerge both general and specific improvements in health.

Final Words

INDIVIDUAL PRACTICE

Understanding that the soma, all that is inside, is expressed bodily is vital to transcending one's patterning. Our lifestyle and occupations, our thoughts and feelings, our character and beliefs, our diet, diseases and surgeries, what we have learned, how we developed, whom we imitated, all of this is expressed in and as the body. Each of us carries and expresses the history of our influences and our reactions to our stressors. They inform and form us. These expressions are visible, sensible to palpation and inwardly perceptible. Seeing how our conditioning affects our functioning provides us with a beginning for self-exploration and can serve our coming to know the nature of our limitations and indicate the way beyond them.

THE BODILY PATTERNS OF EFFORT, ANXIETY, PROTECTION AND COLLAPSE

Thomas Hanna observed that what he called the bodily pattern of effort is focused in the extensor and abductor systems especially through the chronic hyper-contraction of the paraspinal musculature. He hypothesized that this pattern derives from the Landau response seen in infants in their beginning efforts to stand and go forth in the world. This pattern radiates outwards from the centre.

The bodily pattern of anxiety is rooted at the vital centre of the body in the chronic over-contraction of the abdominal musculature. According to Feldenkrais, this pattern begins with the startle reflex observable in infants' self-protective reflex reaction to the threats of falling and loud noises. This pattern radiates outwards from the centre.

The bodily pattern of collapse is rooted in the collapse of the centre of the body whereby inadequate compensations have to be made globally to organize movement in the actural dynamic.

The bodily pattern of protection is focused at any place of injury and derives from the habituation of the trauma reflex. That pattern radiates outwards from that place and is refracted through the axis of the body. The trauma reflex is stimulated at the spinal cord level in response to an injury, trauma or even surgery. Responding to such an event the nervous system stimulates muscular contraction at and around the trauma site to protect and splint the injured area in order to give the metabolic processes time to heal the damage. If this splinting is not consciously or consistently released once the healing period is past, a habit of muscular splinting may develop, pain associated with the injury may not disappear as a consequence, and together these occurrences may cause the rest of the body to adapt to the splinting or the pain. These adaptations are accomplished by pulling away from the pain or by balancing the contraction surrounding the place of injury via a contraction elsewhere in the system through the central axis. Such adaptations, in becoming chronic themselves, may prolong pain or create new pains.

The problem with these patterns, unlike learned responses that have become habitual, is their reflexive nature wherein there is no memory of their origin. Learned patterns on the other hand that have become subcortical are, as Larry Goldfarb has joked, patterns that one has forgotten and then forgotten that one has forgotten.

Pain itself is not necessarily the indication of the place of a trauma. This is another reason addressing pain directly may not be effective in resolving it. Pain is an effect. The cause, which may be far from the site of any pain, must be undone to undo the pain. Indeed pain, especially in cases of trauma, often results from a complex interaction of established patterns with a triggering event. A further problem relative to the resolution of chronic pain is that the neural pathways to the brain may be so habituated to firing that an inconsequential triggering event can re-stimulate the reaction pattern or chronic pain response.

When an injury has been severe enough to damage the person, a short or long period of time needs to be allowed for the natural processes to heal that hurt before any address may be made to any reactions to the trauma. As soon as it can be helpful after that healing is completed those reactions should be addressed, or months or years in the future the person can begin to manifest inexplicable signs which have their source in that initial natural reflex reaction and are only efforts by the person to balance or compensate for that reaction.

It is interesting to consider how Alexander and Feldenkrais perhaps exemplified in themselves the pattern of effort in Alexander's case and of anxiety in that of Feldenkrais. Alexander was the eldest son, probably cultured to a British Empire psyche – 'stiff upper lip, chin up, shoulders back, chest out', all of which would shorten and narrow the back and pull the head back and down on the neck in a particular way. He set off to Australia and later England to seek his fame and fortune, and responded with a defamation suit when libelled in South Africa. All of this suggests a personality who perceived the world in terms of challenges. Alexander focused on the expansion of the back in its two dimensions of length and width rather than the expansion of the trunk in its three dimensions of length, width and depth, the pushing forward (and apparent deepening) of the trunk being one of the signs, according to Hanna, of the bodily pattern of effort.

Feldenkrais, on the other hand, was a member of a threatened minority, made his own way across war-torn Europe at a young age to Palestine, often carried survival-oriented gadgets with him, had a special interest in defense and the martial arts, focused on anxiety as the primary psycho-emotional problem in his first book on his method, *Body and Mature Behaviour*, and advocated compensating for felt deficiencies – all of which suggests a personality who perceived the world in terms of threats and who took remedial counteraction.

As an aside, the essence of the suit brought by Alexander against the South African doctor who had libelled him was Alexander's objection to the doctor's statement that Alexander claimed that through the Technique one could learn to control directly any part of the body like a machine. This is a fundamental misunderstanding of the nature of the 'control' sought in the Technique, which brings the individual via the resolution of habit to a place of freedom, which renewed freedom allows the individual to find the most effective manner of action. It is perhaps a consequence of Alexander's poor choice of the word 'control' in the title of his book, *Constructive Conscious Control of the Individual*, and in his designation of the organization of human movement in the actural dynamic as 'the primary control' rather than, perhaps, 'the primary coordination'.

Even if a person could come to control any part of him- or herself in such a manner, apart from learning Ouled Nail dance, this wouldn't serve the organization of function, which is a global process. The so-called primary control involves the dynamics and coordination of the relationship of the head with the neck and of the head–neck relationship with the back and, via the centre, with the rest of the body and, via the pelvis and legs, with the ground. As more and more of that functional gestalt is apprehended the freer the person is to effectively access movement in accordance with his or her intentions.

FREEDOM IN ACTION

The goal of the Alexander Technique and of somatic methods in general is freedom in action. The means to this end are, 'from the outside', refined manipulation and, 'from the inside', the use of conscious intelligence.

Alexander once wrote that freedom is a plane to be reached. Paradoxically freedom must also be the way of 'arriving' there. The use and practice of awareness, intelligence, inhibition and direction are signs and means of freedom. The results in time of such freedom in the use of the self are pleasure, balance, effectiveness and lightness. On that foundation a thief can become a better thief, a dancer, a better dancer, and a good person, a better one.

In *Still Life with Woodpecker*, Tom Robbins creates the cleverest of images. On a pack of Camel cigarettes, the word 'choice' appears in 'choice Virginia tobacco'. When one turns the package to a mirror all the images and words except for the word 'choice' are reversed. Remarkably this is actually so. The message from the universe is clear: the fact of choice remains unaltered in every dimension. Thomas Hanna emphasized that, in order to grasp somatic methods, you have to 'walk through the looking glass' – that is, you have to make a paradigm shift. One thing that will not change in the new paradigm is the requirement to choose intelligently now and now and now.

The justification for any treatise designed to communicate an understanding of the Alexander Technique is that such an understanding will serve an improved manner of action. I hope this elaboration of the method and its principles and practices encourages you to undertake such a journey of self-discovery.

References

Alexander, F.M. (2000) *The Universal Constant in Living* (ed. Jean Fischer). London: Mouritz.

Alexander, F.M. (2001) *The Use of the Self.* London: Orion.

Alexander, F.M. (2004) *Constructive Conscious Control of the Individual.* London: Mouritz.

Binkley, G. (1993) *The Expanding Self: How the Alexander Technique Changed My Life.* STAT Books.

Feldenkrais, M. (1950) *Body and Mature Behaviour.* New York, NY: International Universities Press.

Harding, D. (2006) *On Having No Head: Zen and the Rediscovery of the Obvious.* Carlsbad, CA: Inner Directions Publishing.

Samraj, Adi Da (1977) *The Paradox of Instruction.* Lower Lake, CA: Dawn Horse Press.

Samraj, Adi Da (1999) *The Ego-'I' is the Illusion of Relatedness.* Lower Lake, CA: Dawn Horse Press.

Schmidt, R. (ed.) (1985) *The Fundamentals of Neurophysiology.* Heidelberg: Springer.

Selye, H. (1978) *The Stress of Life.* London: McGraw-Hill.

Westfeldt, L. (1998) *F. Matthias Alexander: The Man and His Work: Memoirs of Training in the Alexander Technique 1931–34.* London: Mouritz.

Recommended Reading

THE ALEXANDER TECHNIQUE

In Conversation with John Nicholls and Sean Carey
John Nicholls
Clear, comprehensive, concise and considered presentation of the Technique

THE RESURRECTION OF THE BODY

F. M. Alexander
Selections, with an excellent introduction by Edward Maisel, the editor

THE USE OF THE SELF

F. M. Alexander
Perhaps Alexander's most accessible and clear book

THE EXPANDING SELF

Goddard Binkley
A most interesting autobiographical account of the author's several years of lessons with Alexander where the 'lessons' learned in F.M.'s lessons are correlated to the latter's writings

AWARENESS THROUGH MOVEMENT

Moshe Feldenkrais
Feldenkrais' introduction to his Method with ATM transcripts with commentary pertaining to movement fundamentals

HIGHER JUDO

Moshe Feldenkrais

Contains Feldenkrais' first rendering of his somatic education method

SOMATICS

Thomas Hanna

Hanna's deceptively simple elaboration of the Feldenkrais Method, Hanna's own work and the field of somatic learning in general

LISTENING TO THE BODY

Robert Masters

Contains a useful introduction to somatic methodology with transcripts of ATMs devised by Masters

Acknowledgments

Thanks to Denis Lynn, Tony Foxton
and Pedro de Alcantara for reading early drafts;
to Denis also for the photography;
to Craig Allen for the original layout and cover design;
David Erland for the illustrations;
Michael Frederick for writing the foreword
and encouraging me to publish;
John Nicholls for his teaching;
and to Jessica Kingsley and the staff at Singing Dragon
for their commitment to high-quality work.

Graeme Lynn has studied and practiced the Alexander Technique and the Feldenkrais Method for more than 30 years. He has trained as well in Hatha yoga and Ida Rolf's structural bodywork and is among a handful of individuals who studied intensively with Thomas Hanna. His continued commitment to the practice of somatic methodology has resulted in successful client-based and personal work in the resolution of functional issues.